Teen Guide to
MANAGING
MENTAL HEALTH

James Roland

AF148763

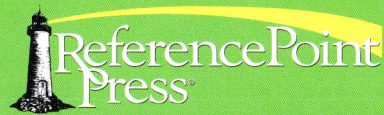

ReferencePoint
Press

San Diego, CA

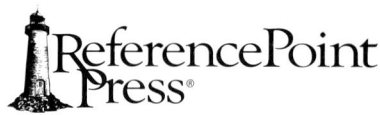

About the Author

After graduating from the University of Oregon, James Roland became a news-paper reporter, primarily focused on education. He later became a magazine writer and editor, as well as an author of more than a dozen books. He and his wife, Heidi, have three children, Chris, Alexa, and Carson.

© 2024 ReferencePoint Press, Inc.
Printed in the United States

For more information, contact:
ReferencePoint Press, Inc.
PO Box 27779
San Diego, CA 92198
www.ReferencePointPress.com

LIBRARY OF CONGRESS CATALOGING-IN-PUBLICATION DATA

Names: Roland, James, author.
Title: Teen guide to managing mental health / by James Roland.
Description: San Diego, CA : ReferencePoint Press, Inc., 2024. | Includes
    bibliographical references and index.
Identifiers: LCCN 2023009833 (print) | LCCN 2023009834 (ebook) | ISBN
    9781678205928 (library binding) | ISBN 9781678205935 (ebook)
Subjects: LCSH: Teenagers--Mental health.
Classification: LCC RJ499 .R642 2024 (print) | LCC RJ499 (ebook) | DDC
    616.8900835--dc23/eng/20230417
LC record available at https://lccn.loc.gov/2023009833
LC ebook record available at https://lccn.loc.gov/2023009834

CONTENTS

Your Mind and You

Selena Gomez, Ryan Reynolds, Simone Biles, and Pete Davidson are among the many celebrities who have become more open about their mental health issues in recent years. Indeed, the list of prominent people who struggle with disorders such as anxiety, depression, bipolar disorder, and substance use disorder seems to grow all the time and includes top athletes like Dallas Cowboys quarterback Dak Prescott and Olympic champion snowboarder Chloe Kim. While such issues were once considered too stigmatizing to share publicly, the increase in mental health problems—particularly among America's youth—has led to more widespread acceptance of open and compassionate discussions around the issue.

After Gomez was diagnosed with bipolar disorder, she gave interviews about her condition and publicly discussed the importance of getting help. She even made a documentary about mental health called *Selena Gomez: My Mind & Me* and has urged young people to treat mental health issues as they would any other concern or problem. The singer-actress also stresses the importance of learning about mental illness, a problem that affects one in six American youths each year, according to the National Alliance on Mental Illness. In a 2022 roundtable discussion on mental health at the White House, Gomez emphasized the value of being open about your emotional and psychological health. "Just talking about your own journey can help," she said. "It sets the example that it's a topic that can and should be discussed freely, and without shame."[1]

A year later, in his State of the Union address, President Joe Biden highlighted the urgency of addressing the rising levels of anxiety and depression among the nation's young people, saying, "Let's do more on mental health, especially for our children. When millions of young people are struggling with bullying, violence, trauma, we owe them greater access to mental health care at school."[2]

Mental Health Education

Although you learn about math, science, history, and other subjects in school, formal curricula don't prioritize learning about or understanding mental health. So it's up to you to learn what good mental health looks like and how to recognize signs of a disorder. Your well-being, or the well-being of someone you care about, may depend on it.

The first thing to know is that mental health concerns exist on a continuum from everyday stress to severe mental illness, and it is important to learn how to manage your mental health because it affects every other part of your life. The second is that everyone follows a different path when it comes to their thoughts, feelings, experiences, and behaviors. For example, relationships with family members, classmates, and teachers may cause emotional and psychological distress for some people, but those relationships may be the keys to stability and happiness for others.

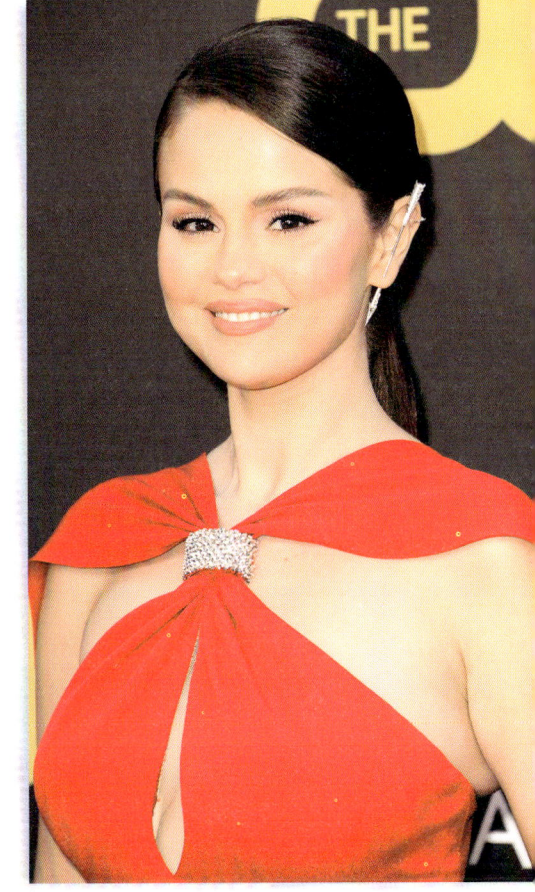

Selena Gomez, pictured at the Annual Critics Choice Awards in 2022, has been open about her struggles with bipolar disorder.

Managing your mental health may require little more than pursuing rewarding activities and living a healthy lifestyle, nourished by supportive relationships and an environment that keeps you grounded, safe, and secure. But if you're like a lot of people, you may need extra help to manage your stress, cope with difficult relationships, and overcome fears or feelings you don't quite understand. Learning tools and strategies to build positive mental health habits can help you succeed in school, work, relationships, and everything else life has to offer.

It is critical to pay close attention to your mental health in adolescence, since research suggests that about half of all mental health disorders first appear before a person turns fourteen, while about 75 percent show up by the time someone is twenty-four. "Recent data has revealed that more kids and teens are dealing with anxiety, depression and difficulty coping with life's daily challenges than ever,"[3] says Cleveland Clinic psychologist Amy Lee.

The more you understand what's going on in your heart and mind, the better able you'll be to meet challenges that arise. Don't be afraid to confront uncomfortable feelings, and be willing to get help if you need it. Exploring your feelings and sharing them with others can be empowering and make things seem less overwhelming and mysterious. No one benefits from keeping their emotions locked inside, especially when it comes to powerful feelings like sadness, hopelessness, fear, and confusion. Those are all normal emotions, no less valid than happiness, hopefulness, or excitement. "You should never stop figuring out who you are," says Gomez. "I just hope that people [who are suffering] know they're not alone."[4]

CHAPTER ONE

The Meaning of Mental Health

Mental health refers to a person's emotional and psychological well-being. It is how you cope with positive and negative emotions, as well as how you view the world. Your mental health also affects how you think and feel about yourself. Your ability to be productive, make good decisions, and set goals are all influenced by the state of your mental health.

Your mental health impacts the way you handle stress, success, disappointments, frustrations, new opportunities, unexpected events, and day-to-day interactions with family, friends, teachers, and others. Signs of good mental health include feeling relatively confident and maintaining an optimistic, positive outlook, as well as having a sense of belonging and keeping a realistic, grounded perspective—even in situations that pose real challenges. "Mental health is the state you are in when your body and mind are collectively working together," explains Royce Lee, an associate professor of psychiatry and behavioral neuroscience at the University of Chicago Medical Center. "A helpful way to think about it is that your brain is working in a way to serve you well."[5]

While it is important to understand what mental health is, it's also helpful to know what it isn't. Mental health is not the complete absence of emotional or psychological distress. You might describe a person with no serious illnesses or injuries as "healthy," even though that individual might occasionally have migraine headaches or need glasses to see at a distance. Similarly, someone could be described as being mentally healthy even if he or she gets claustrophobic in a crowd, is occasionally moody, or sometimes loses sleep worrying about final exams or climate change. Psychologist Lisa Damour, author of *The Emotional Lives of Teenagers*, told the *New York Times* in 2023 that mental health is often incorrectly characterized as only "feeling good, happy, calm or relaxed," when in reality it is "about having feelings that fit the moment—even if those feelings are unwanted or painful—and managing them in effective ways."[6] In other words, feeling sad after a breakup or after failing a test is an appropriate emotional response and can indicate good mental health. However, feeling sad for no discernible reason or in circumstances that would normally lend themselves to feeling happy could be a sign that your mental health might need some attention.

The Difference Between Mental Health and Mental Illness

The terms *mental health* and *mental illness* are sometimes used interchangeably, as though they mean the same thing. This isn't the case, but they are related. Mental health comprises your overall emotional, psychological, and social well-being, but it exists on a spectrum. You can have "good" mental health days when you feel especially happy, are calm, and your self-esteem is strong. Then you can have days when you feel stressed, overwhelmed, or just plain blue.

Mental illness is much different from having a bad day or a bad week. A mental illness, also known as a mental health disorder, is a defined medical issue that can be diagnosed on the basis of whether a person meets certain criteria. It can be treated with some combination of psychotherapy (talk therapy), medication, and lifestyle changes. "Everyone has mental health, just like everyone has physical health," explains Stan Preston, a mental health program manager at Misericordia Community Hospital in

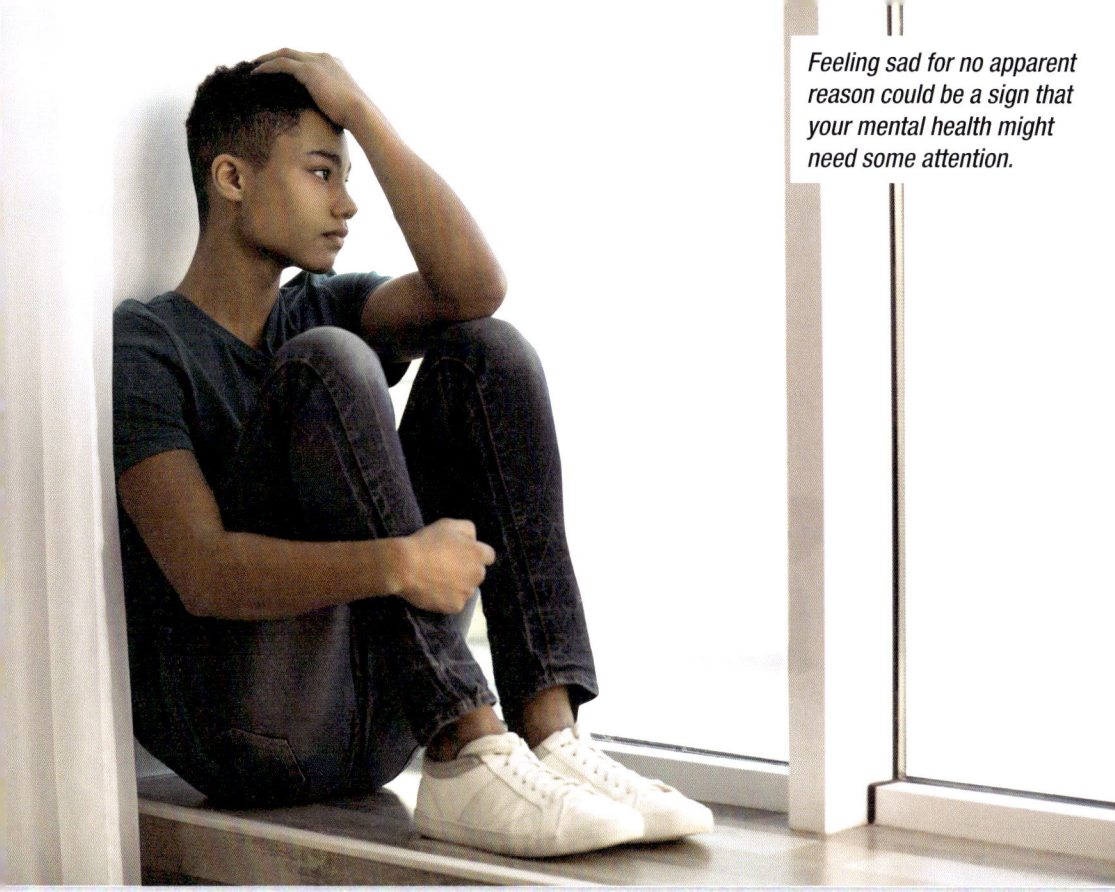

Feeling sad for no apparent reason could be a sign that your mental health might need some attention.

Edmonton, Canada. "Not everyone will experience mental illness, but everyone will have periods of time when they struggle with their mental well-being, just as we have physical health issues from time to time."[7]

A key difference between a mental health concern and an illness is that the latter often interferes with your ability to function or carry out your daily responsibilities over time. It is normal, for example, to feel stressed on a particular day, but mentally healthy individuals are still able to finish their homework or enjoy time with their friends. Having bipolar disorder or another mental health disorder, however, can make it difficult just to get out of bed in the morning.

Understanding the difference between mental illness and mental health may offer you perspective on your own feelings. Recognizing the differences can help you figure out whether you (or a friend or relative) are experiencing a temporary change in mood or are displaying signs of a more serious condition.

Everyone Is Dealing with Something

When you see people who come across as happy and successful or otherwise appear to be cruising through life, it may be tempting to assume that they have achieved optimal mental health and well-being. But the truth is, everybody is dealing with something. On any given day, it might be something minor, like a disappointing report card or an argument with a friend. But even the seemingly happiest and most successful people often have serious struggles that they don't let others see. In fact, clinical psychologist Jonathan Schaefer suggests that the often-quoted estimate that one in five people have some type of mental health disorder is far too low; in his experience, more than 80 percent of the population is dealing with some type of mental health challenge. His advice for young people: "Prepare them for the fact that their friends and their future partners will probably have some of these issues, and that's okay. Most of the time they're temporary, and they happen to almost everyone."

Quoted in Seth Gillihan, "Mental Illness Is Far More 'Normal' than We Think," *Psychology Today*, May 17, 2021. www.psychologytoday.com.

Types of Mental Health Disorders

A mental health disorder is a medical condition that affects your emotions, thoughts, and behaviors. These disorders take many forms, and their related symptoms have many degrees of severity. For example, you can have a mild anxiety disorder that is troubling but does not interfere with your ability to go to school or participate in daily activities. A severe anxiety disorder, however, may make it difficult to be out in public or manage routine responsibilities.

There are more than two hundred classified mental health disorders, but three of them—anxiety disorder, depression, and posttraumatic stress disorder (PTSD)—make up nearly one-third of all mental illness diagnoses in the United States. Among teens, anxiety and depression are by far the most commonly diagnosed mental health disorders, though an estimated 3 to 15 percent of girls and 1 to 6 percent of boys develop PTSD.

Anxiety Disorder

Characterized by excessive worry and tension, anxiety can also cause physical changes such as increased heart rate and difficulty catching your breath. Everybody experiences anxiety from time to time, but it usually subsides, say, after taking your driving test or finishing a speech. This type of anxiety is usually focused on a specific event or threat and is thus short lived.

However, when a person has an anxiety disorder, their symptoms don't disappear and can actually worsen over time. The worries that accompany an anxiety disorder tend to be associated with past or future events and may be difficult for an individual to define or explain. Dr. Leana Wen, a health policy professor at the George Washington University Milken Institute School for Public Health, says:

> It's crucial to distinguish feelings of anxiety from the medical diagnosis of an anxiety disorder. Anxiety is a normal reaction to stress. Everyone feels some level of nervousness to situations in their lives. Anxiety disorders are characterized by a persistent, excessive fear or anxiety that affects a person's ability to function. They can lead to people avoiding situations—social engagements, professional functions, appointments or even daily errands for example—and affecting their jobs, education, and personal relationships.[8]

People who suffer from an anxiety disorder may also have intrusive, repetitive, unpleasant, or scary thoughts. These are frequently unrealistic or exaggerated, so anxiety disorder treatment typically emphasizes strategies that help people replace unhelpful thoughts with more reasonable or constructive ones. With practice, such treatment can significantly improve a person's quality of life.

> "It's crucial to distinguish feelings of anxiety from the medical diagnosis of an anxiety disorder."[8]
>
> —Leana Wen, George Washington University health policy professor

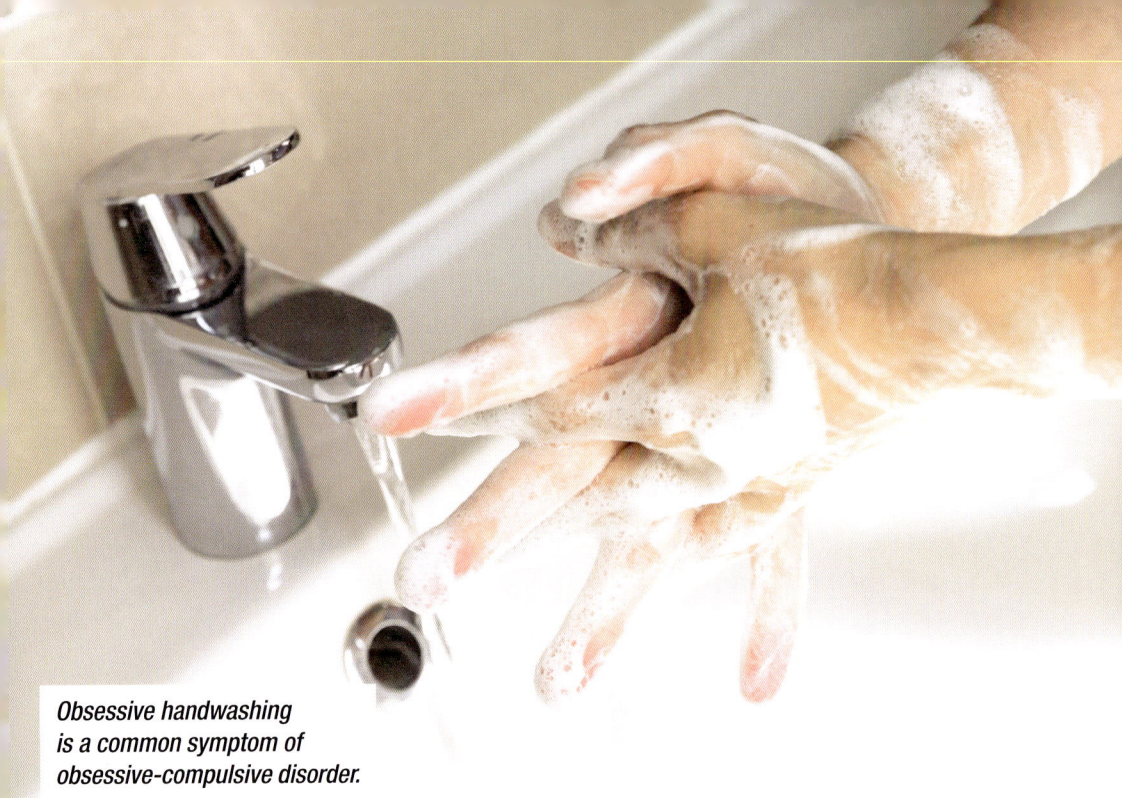

Obsessive handwashing is a common symptom of obsessive-compulsive disorder.

For this reason, Dr. Daniel Pine, a National Institutes of Health neuroscientist and psychiatrist, says, "Anxiety disorders are one of the most treatable mental health problems we see."[9]

Under the broad umbrella of "anxiety disorder," there are several subtypes: generalized anxiety disorder (GAD), obsessive-compulsive disorder (OCD), panic disorder, and social anxiety disorder. GAD is characterized by chronic and excessive worry and tension, often with nothing to trigger it. GAD is similar to other anxiety disorders in some ways, but people with GAD tend to experience an overwhelming sense of anxiety that is ill defined, or they skip from one anxiety to another throughout the day. GAD-related anxieties are often based on real-world situations but the worst-case scenarios of these.

OCD is characterized by recurring and intrusive thoughts (obsessions) that are often frightening or upsetting and/or

> "Anxiety disorders are one of the most treatable mental health problems we see."[9]
>
> —Daniel Pine, National Institutes of Health neuroscientist and psychiatrist

repetitive behaviors (compulsions), such as washing and rewashing your hands, checking and rechecking that a door is locked, or frequently arranging items on a desk. The intrusive thoughts may or may not be based on realistic fears. The compulsions are rituals believed to prevent what the anxious mind fears will happen if they are not done. Sometimes the compulsions provide temporary relief, while not doing them can make the anxiety worse.

Someone with a panic disorder experiences unpredictable and repeated episodes of panic or fear along with physical symptoms such as heart palpitations, chest pain, shortness of breath, and nausea. Having one or two panicky episodes throughout your life is normal, but if these attacks occur more often or you experience long stretches of time fearing your next one, you may have a panic disorder.

Finally, social anxiety disorder, also known as social phobia, is characterized by overwhelming anxiety and self-consciousness in situations involving other people. The disorder may present symptoms in everyday circumstances, such as being in a store or other public place, eating in front of others, sitting in class, giving a speech, or performing in an athletic or theatrical setting.

Depression

Depression considered serious enough to be diagnosed as an illness is also called major depressive disorder or clinical depression. Depression causes sad, hopeless feelings, and individuals often withdraw from people and activities they used to enjoy or find fulfilling. Someone who is clinically depressed may experience depressive episodes, which last for at least two weeks and are dominated by low mood, feelings of worthlessness, drastic changes in sleep patterns, and pain or other physical ailments that can't be explained.

When she was thirteen years old, Brooklyn Williams, a student in western Pennsylvania, lost her mother to breast cancer. Months later, in the spring of 2020, the COVID-19 pandemic and the shift to remote learning further upended her world, leaving her numb, sad, and struggling to get through each day. When in-school learning resumed that fall, Williams tried to put up a strong front before her friends, teachers, and family. "I was putting everyone else first, and making sure they saw me as a happy person," she said in 2022. But before long, Williams developed severe digestive problems and had difficulty getting out of bed and through the school day. She began to question whether life was worth living. "I was going through it alone, but once I reached out, things went from zero to one hundred really fast,"[10] she explained, adding that once her father and her best friend understood what she was going through, she began therapy and started the healing process.

Later, in high school, Williams founded the Chill Club, an after-school club that included yoga, crafts, and other stress management activities to help kids going through whatever challenges they faced. "I thought, 'If this is making me feel better, then maybe it will make others feel better too.'"[11] Williams shared her experience with members of Congress at a 2022 hearing on adolescent mental health.

Anyone can experience depression, and it is not always clear what causes it. Scientists believe that several factors can play a role, including structural differences in the brain and an imbalance of certain brain chemicals, such as neurotransmitters (e.g., dopamine, serotonin, norepinephrine), which carry messages between neurons. Hormonal imbalances may also play a role. Having a family history of depression can raise a person's risk of developing the same condition, so research is ongoing to identify gene mutations that may account for inherited cases.

Various risk factors have also been identified as possibly contributing to whether a person develops depression. Experiencing any type of trauma—such as physical, sexual, or emotional abuse—the loss of a loved one, or serious financial or health hardship can trigger depression in a person. Those with a history of alcohol or drug abuse, as well as those with certain personality traits such as having low self-esteem or a pessimistic or fixed outlook, are also more prone to depression.

The Language of Mental Health

It is common for people to describe someone who is especially detail oriented as "a little OCD" or a cautious person as having "anxiety." The casual use of these psychological terms can be harmful, however. Labeling someone as having a mental health disorder without that person receiving a diagnosis can create a false perception that affects how the person thinks, feels, and behaves. Tossing around terms like *depressed* or *bipolar* may also trivialize the seriousness of those conditions.

Conversely, as noted by journalist Maia Szalavitz, hearing people use phrases like "I'm a little OCD" can sometimes be helpful. It underscores the idea that mental health disorders can have a range of symptom severity and that many people tend toward one condition or another. It's just important to understand what these conditions really mean and to avoid stereotypes. In a *New York Times* column, Szalavitz writes, "The more we recognize that we all have traits that at the extremes can be disabling, the more compassionate we will be and the more we will be able to benefit from everyone's talents."

Maia Szalavitz, "I Don't Mind If You Say You Have 'a Little OCD,'" *New York Times*, January 22, 2023. www.nytimes.com.

Certain populations are particularly vulnerable to developing depression. For example, members of the LGBTQ+ community also experience depression at higher rates than the general public. According to the Trevor Project's 2022 National Survey on LGBTQ Youth Mental Health, 58 percent of LGBTQ youth experience symptoms of depression, compared to an estimated 3 percent of youths in the general population.

PTSD

PTSD can develop after experiencing or witnessing a frightening, violent, or extremely upsetting event. It may also result from episodes of emotional abuse or prolonged emotional trauma. PTSD is a mental health disorder characterized by flashbacks, nightmares, severe anxiety, and uncontrollable and intrusive thoughts related to the trauma.

Traumatic events that may trigger PTSD include childhood abuse and/or neglect, sexual and/or physical assault, automobile accidents, military combat, human-made or natural disasters, the death of a loved one, or another extreme emotional challenge. In recent years the COVID-19 pandemic, school shootings (whether witnessed firsthand or followed in news coverage), and natural disasters like hurricanes and massive wildfires have only intensified the emotional challenges facing young people. "These kids have been through the wringer," says Brittney Schrick, a family life specialist and assistant professor at the University of Arkansas. "It's really hard to be a teenager right now. I think all we can do as future employers, as parents, as aunts and uncles, and mentors, is keep in mind that they're going to need some help, and it doesn't make them weak, bad or lazy. They need support and grace."[12]

Other Mental Health Disorders

Anxiety, depression, and PTSD represent a large share of the mental health disorders diagnosed every year, but many other mental illnesses affect millions of people around the world. Some of these disorders first appear when people are in their teens, while others may not develop until later in life.

Bipolar disorder, for example, is usually diagnosed in a person's late teens or early twenties. Bipolar disorder is characterized by severe mood swings ranging from depressive (low) phases to manic (high) phases, with each phase lasting days or months at a time and marked by some potentially harmful symptoms and behaviors. The National Institute of Mental Health estimates that about 2.9 percent of teens have bipolar disorder and that the condition is slightly more common among females than males.

Eating disorders, however, are nearly twice as likely to affect females as males, with nearly 4 percent of adolescent girls experiencing some type of eating disorder. Health experts estimate that a much higher percentage of teens, especially girls, experience occasional or frequent episodes of disordered eating that may not necessarily be considered diagnosable. There are several different

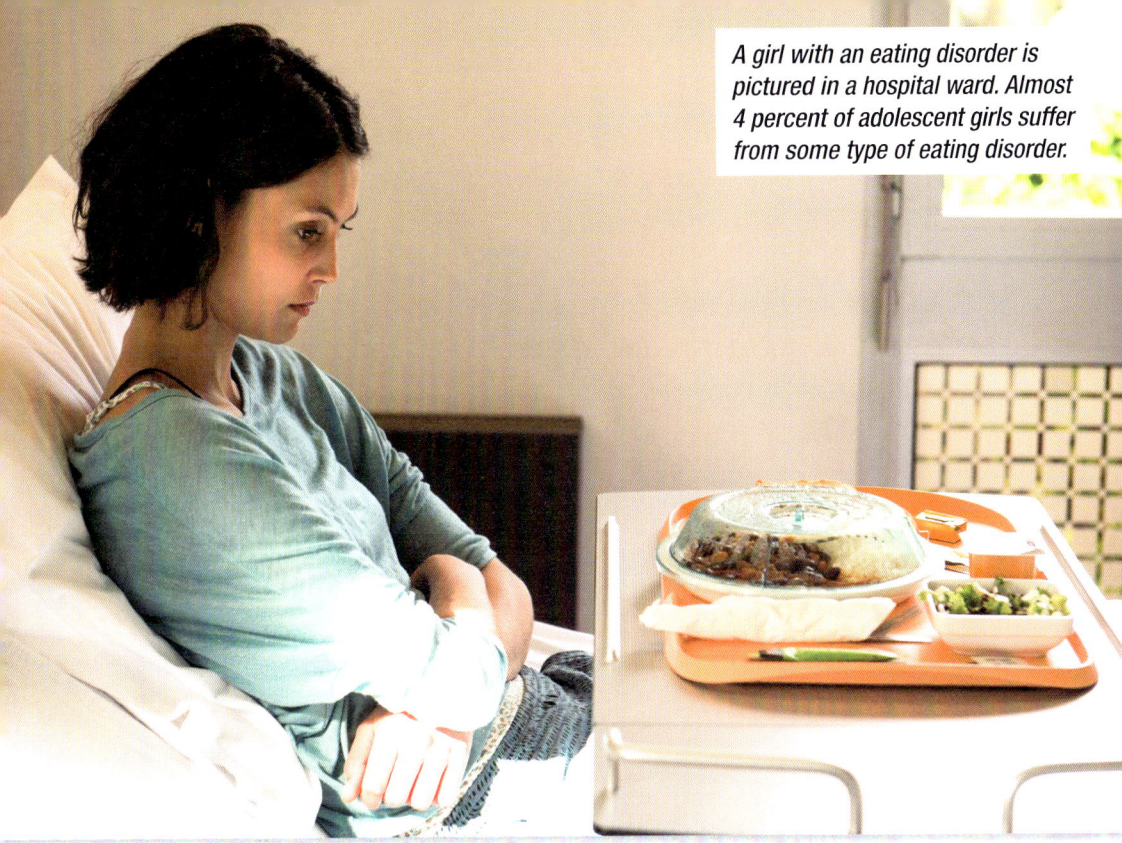

A girl with an eating disorder is pictured in a hospital ward. Almost 4 percent of adolescent girls suffer from some type of eating disorder.

types of eating disorders, including anorexia nervosa and bulimia, though they all involve disturbances in eating patterns and behaviors and are related to intrusive or upsetting thoughts and feelings.

For Michigan high school volleyball player Amelia Haywood, the isolation that marked the COVID-19 pandemic led her to overly focus on exercise and food—the few things in life she could control. Soon she started eating less and less, and in 2021 she was hospitalized for an eating disorder that was leaving her malnourished, weak, and in need of emergency medical care and counseling. Before that first trip to the hospital, her mother asked the listless, formerly energetic teen what was going on. Haywood told her she was struggling with food. "That was probably the hardest thing I've ever said in my whole entire life," she later told Michigan Radio. Haywood eventually got the treatment she needed and is back to feeling healthy and happy again. "For people who are struggling, just know that it gets better. The really hard time is temporary," Haywood said. "I'm six months out, and I am starting to get activity back [in my life.] So I can hang out with my friends and live my life how I want to live. And I know it's really hard to recover, and really hard to reach out. But at the end of the day, it's so worth it."[13]

Just as an eating disorder represents an unhealthy relationship with food, a substance use disorder involves an unhealthy and potentially dangerous relationship with prescription medications, alcohol, or other drugs. *Substance use disorder* can refer to frequent abuse of alcohol or drugs or to addiction, which is a psychological and/or physical dependence on alcohol or other drugs.

Schizophrenia is another mental health disorder, one that can be especially challenging to treat. It is characterized by an abnormal interpretation of reality, hallucinations, delusions, and illogical thoughts and behaviors that can severely interfere with everyday functioning.

Recognizing Good Mental Health

While it is helpful to know the signs and characteristics of mental illness, it is equally important to know what good mental health feels and looks like. Good mental health can allow a person to be productive and resilient (having the ability to adapt to stress, challenges, and changes). Good mental health is also associated with healthy relationships and self-esteem, as well as the ability to experience feelings of happiness, compassion, optimism, and empathy.

The better you are able to recognize what constitutes the difference between good mental health and a mental health disorder, the more quickly you will be able to help yourself or others get help before the struggle becomes overwhelming.

CHAPTER TWO

Factors That Affect Mental Health

There are many factors that affect a teen's mental health. Some stem from home and family life, as well as the influence of peers, school, the media, and other external forces. Your genetics and brain chemistry also significantly determine your mental health and your risk for diseases and disorders. Finally, your physical health is directly tied to your emotional and psychological well-being.

Basic needs, such as eating a good diet and getting sufficient sleep, lay the foundation for good mental health. Getting regular exercise, being outdoors, pursuing hobbies, having an emotionally supportive family, and developing positive relationships with other people further support mental health. Of course, a person can have all of these things going for him or her and still occasionally struggle emotionally and psychologically. "A mental illness is not always the result of childhood experiences," explains Cleveland Clinic psychologist Scott Bea. "Some people have wonderful home environments and amazing caregivers, but still experience a mental health disorder."[14]

When a person who is genetically disposed to mental illness also has other negative or unhealthy factors present, he or she may face even greater risks of chronic stress and long-term psychological challenges. Food or housing insecurity, abuse or neglect at home, trauma, and other types of adversity often befall those who struggle with many mental health risk factors, and these experiences whittle away at their sense of well-being. Understanding the conditions and factors that can threaten your mental health may allow you to see what is at the root of your struggles or what troubles might lie ahead if your problems go unaddressed.

The Teenage Brain

Perhaps you have found yourself wondering why your emotions are all over the place or why some feelings seem particularly overwhelming. Know that you are in good company among other teenagers. In fact, you have a lot in common with the youth of other animal species, too! In humans and other animals, the brain is actually the last organ to fully mature. The human brain continues to develop into the mid-twenties.

Until then, your brain is primarily wired for learning and memory formation. The regions of the brain responsible for decision-making, impulse control, judgment, and empathy are among the last to develop. That's why children and teenagers often make decisions based on emotions, which are controlled largely by the brain's amygdala and limbic system. Once the frontal lobes—which handle higher-level thinking, reason, and planning—are fully developed, they will take over much of the decision-making responsibilities.

Because the adolescent mind is so influenced by emotion, it is more vulnerable to emotional distress. Neurologist Frances Jensen explains that the imbalance between emotions and rational, logical thought in the teenage brain increases the stress response. "This is a concern because too much stress in the teen years changes the way your brain develops," says Jensen. "It can actually set up neurochemical imbalances that increase your risk for depression later in life."[15] This is why stress manage-

20

ment is so important for young people—not just to improve their quality of life in the moment but also to prevent long-term mental health problems.

Brain chemistry is also a major factor regulating emotions and mental health in general. Conditions such as depression, anxiety, and others are rooted in having abnormal levels of various hormones and brain chemicals called neurotransmitters, which act as messengers between cells. Unhealthy levels of dopamine, serotonin, and other neurotransmitters can trigger changes in mood and have other impacts on health. Some people take medication to regulate these levels, but for many others, medication is just one part of the solution. Stress reduction through therapy, meditation, exercise, or other means can also have a powerful influence on brain chemical levels.

Socialization and Isolation

The people with whom you interact, and how often you interact with others, can have a major impact—both good and bad—

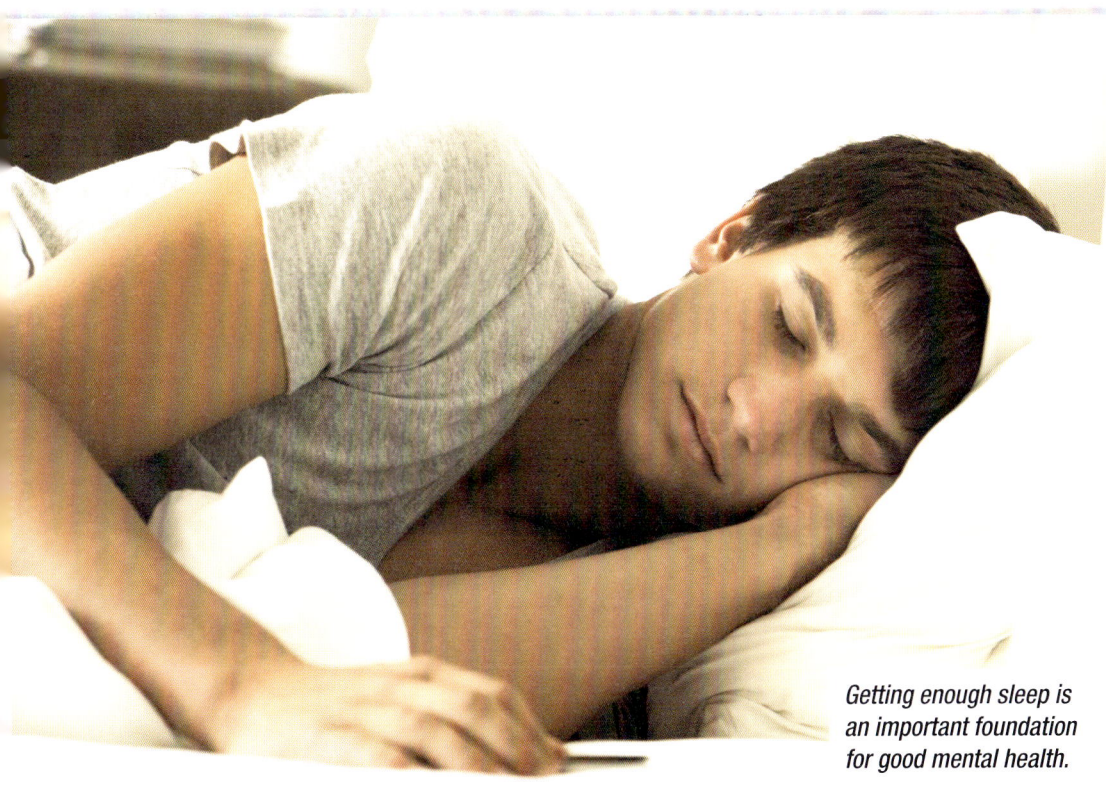

Getting enough sleep is an important foundation for good mental health.

on your mental health. Positive social interactions with friends and loved ones help prevent isolation and can reduce feelings of loneliness.

Though they are similar, loneliness and isolation are distinct in important ways. Loneliness is an internal sense, a subjective feeling of being alone, whether you are physically by yourself or in a room full of people. In fact, recent studies suggest that living in a crowded, urban setting is associated with higher levels of loneliness, while more frequent contact with nature (parks and other green spaces) is associated with lower levels of loneliness. In addition, loneliness is not the same as being alone. You may be quite content sitting alone in your room sometimes listening to music, reading a book, playing video games, or otherwise being occupied with your own thoughts.

Lacking Purpose Affects Your Mental Health

While factors such as family discord or academic struggles are readily identifiable causes of stress, discouragement, or hopelessness, there is another cause that is often overlooked, especially among teens: having a sense of purpose. In psychological terms, purpose is having meaningful and fulfilling goals and responsibilities.

How a sense of purpose affects adolescents' well-being was the subject of a study led by Kaylin Ratner, an educational psychology professor at the University of Illinois. The results, published in 2023, found that teens with a strong sense of purpose had more positive emotions and fewer negative emotions than their peers who scored lower on surveys of purpose. "Importantly, we found that on the days when these adolescents felt more purposeful than usual, they also tended to experience greater well-being," she told the University of Illinois News Bureau. A sense of purpose can be fostered by focusing on career or college plans, volunteering to help others, and being part of a team working toward athletic, artistic, or academic goals. It is also helpful to stop and think about the important role you play in the lives of your friends and family.

Quoted in Sharita Forrest, "A Sense of Purpose May Have Significant Impact on Teens' Emotional Well-Being," News Bureau, February 13, 2023. https://news.illinois.edu.

Isolation, sometimes referred to in psychological terms as "social isolation," is a lack of consistent interaction with other people. People need human contact to thrive, and without it, emotional and psychological health can suffer, as can critical-thinking skills and other important brain functions.

During the COVID-19 pandemic, social isolation presented people of all ages with severe psychological challenges, including high levels of loneliness. Many students attended school remotely and had fewer in-person encounters with friends, peers, coaches, teachers, and other influential people, which led to a spike in reports of anxiety and depression among school-age kids. Therapist Caroline Fenkel notes that social isolation is a major cause of depressive symptoms such as hopelessness, fatigue, and loneliness. "Social isolation can be voluntary or involuntary, short-term or long-term—and the longer isolation lasts, the harder it can be to overcome,"[16] she says, adding that prolonged isolation can make even the thought of social interaction a source of anxiety for teens. It can be easy to get into the habit of saying no to invitations or otherwise avoiding contact with others. But good mental health relies on having regular (daily or weekly) interactions with friends, classmates, family members, neighbors, and other influential individuals.

Family Function

Stable and nurturing family relationships can bolster a teen's mental health while providing a secure home environment and emotional support and guidance. But family environments in which stress levels are high or those characterized by factors such as divorce, domestic violence, drug or alcohol abuse, poverty, and unhealthy relationships are likely to undercut a person's well-being.

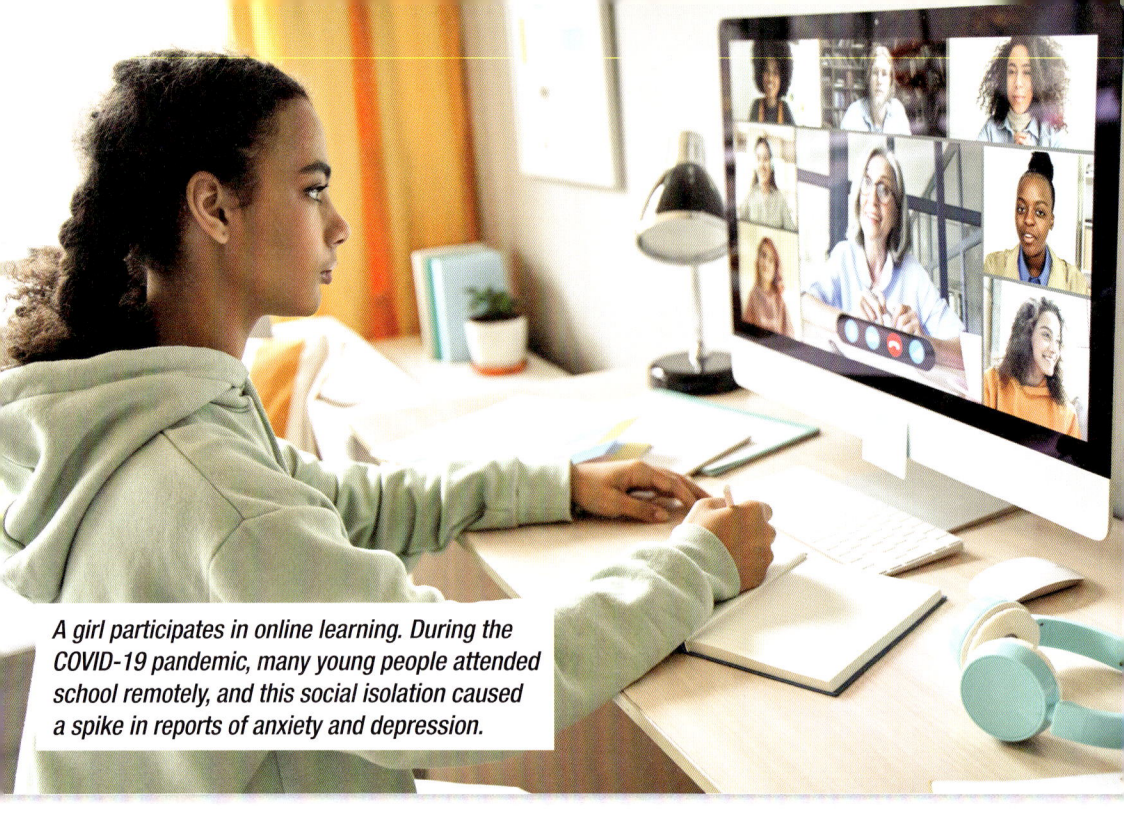

A girl participates in online learning. During the COVID-19 pandemic, many young people attended school remotely, and this social isolation caused a spike in reports of anxiety and depression.

A 2022 study published in the journal *Frontiers in Psychology* found that family dysfunction significantly raises the risk of adolescent depression, while family cohesion—the ability to maintain healthy emotional bonds even in the face of change and challenges—offers teens some protection against depression and other mood disorders. It can be difficult to approach your parents about trouble in the home, but if you let them know how much certain circumstances are upsetting you, it could be the first of many helpful conversations. If you are afraid of talking to your parents, for whatever reason, consider talking with a teacher, school nurse, guidance counselor, or perhaps another relative such as an aunt or uncle.

Social Media

Connecting with friends and expressing yourself creatively are some of the positive benefits offered by social media, but they are hardly the only impacts of using Instagram, TikTok, and other platforms. Social media is also used by teens to bully peers and casually dash off insults and critiques that leave their targets wounded. Research suggests that teens, particularly girls, are uniquely sensitive to insults and criticisms leveled over social media. An internal review by Instagram, for example, found that while most teen users had generally positive experiences with the app, one-third of teenage girls said it made them feel worse about themselves—and yet most had a hard time resisting logging on. A University of Pennsylvania study found that young adults who limited their social media usage to ten minutes a day reported feeling less depressed and lonely than teens who used it more.

Many health experts acknowledge that the "culture of comparison" that exists among young social media consumers poses a real threat to kids who may already have self-esteem issues or other mental health challenges. Cate, a high school student in Washington, told the *Today Show* that her body image struggles were made worse by seeing girls with "perfect bodies" on social media. "I thought, 'Maybe fixing my body will make me feel happier and better,'" she said. Over time, she eventually began dealing with her body image in a healthier way, but she still worries about getting "likes" on Instagram. "I feel like I have to take a post down if it doesn't get enough likes or comments. It makes me wonder if people don't like that post,"[17] she added.

Likewise, for many teenagers, there are few more stressful feelings than the fear of missing out, or FOMO, the sense that other people are having fun without you. FOMO causes people to obsessively check social media, feel negatively about their own life, or become mentally exhausted trying to keep up with others. Anne Marie Albano, director of the Columbia University Clinic for Anxiety and Related Disorders, says that spending a lot of time online promotes problems such as being cyberbullied, romanticizing other people's experiences, or generally feeling disconnected to the outside world. These tendencies only further exacerbate the negative influences that social media has on teens' mental health—and ironically, can cause them to spend even more time online. "There are youth, especially those with social anxiety or depression, who

Gender Identity, Sexual Orientation, and Mental Health Risks

Despite recent advances in LGBTQ representation in mass media and other corners of society, some troubling statistics persist. Members of the LGBTQ community are more than twice as likely as heterosexual individuals to experience mental health issues. Transgender individuals are at even greater risk. They may be up to four times as likely as non-transgender individuals to be diagnosed with a mental health disorder.

Among the many factors that contribute to these numbers are discrimination, family rejection, and harassment, often resulting in violence. "Like with any identity, feeling different—or worse, unaccepted as you are—is a significant risk factor for mental health struggles," says Anna Docherty, an assistant professor of psychiatry at the University of Utah's Huntsman Mental Health Institute. She adds that while most people rely on social support to get through various emotional or psychological challenges, such support can be harder to find for young people struggling with or questioning their gender identity or sexual orientation. If you are in such a situation, try to build a supportive network by opening up to family members and close friends. You may also find help with the GSA Network, which helps students establish GSA clubs in schools and local communities.

Quoted in Leann Bentley, "Why Does the LGBTQIA+ Community Suffer from Poor Mental Health at Higher Rates?," University of Utah Health, July 7, 2021. https://healthcare.utah.edu.

may have a tendency to spend more time online and reduce their real, face-to-face contact with other folks,"[18] says Albano.

Other Mental Health Influences

Among the most common and influential factors that affect a teen's mental health is peer pressure, which can be either a positive or negative force. Kids are well-served by having friends who encourage them to try harder in school or otherwise keep up with healthy, positive, creative activities. Unfortunately, peer pressure often goes the other direction and leads to reckless, risk-taking behavior or bullying. The results can be lower self-esteem or even thoughts of self-harm and suicide.

Mass media also has an enormous impact on teens' mental health. The images shown on television, online and print ads, and social media can both present uplifting and aspirational goals and send extremely dispiriting messages. The National Eating Disorders Association reports that as early as elementary school, the majority of girls have a sense of what an ideal body shape is from mass media, and nearly half say such images make them want to lose weight. Similarly, mass media representations of muscular men or superheroes appear to lead to body dissatisfaction among a sizable number of boys.

The school environment can also have a positive or negative effect on a teen's mental health. School experiences can range from inspiring to tedious to stressful. For some students, the hour they spend in drama class or at basketball practice can help motivate them to make it through the less pleasant parts of the school day. Other students might love everything about school, while still others might struggle to find anything interesting about school. If school feels like a negative factor in your life, talk with

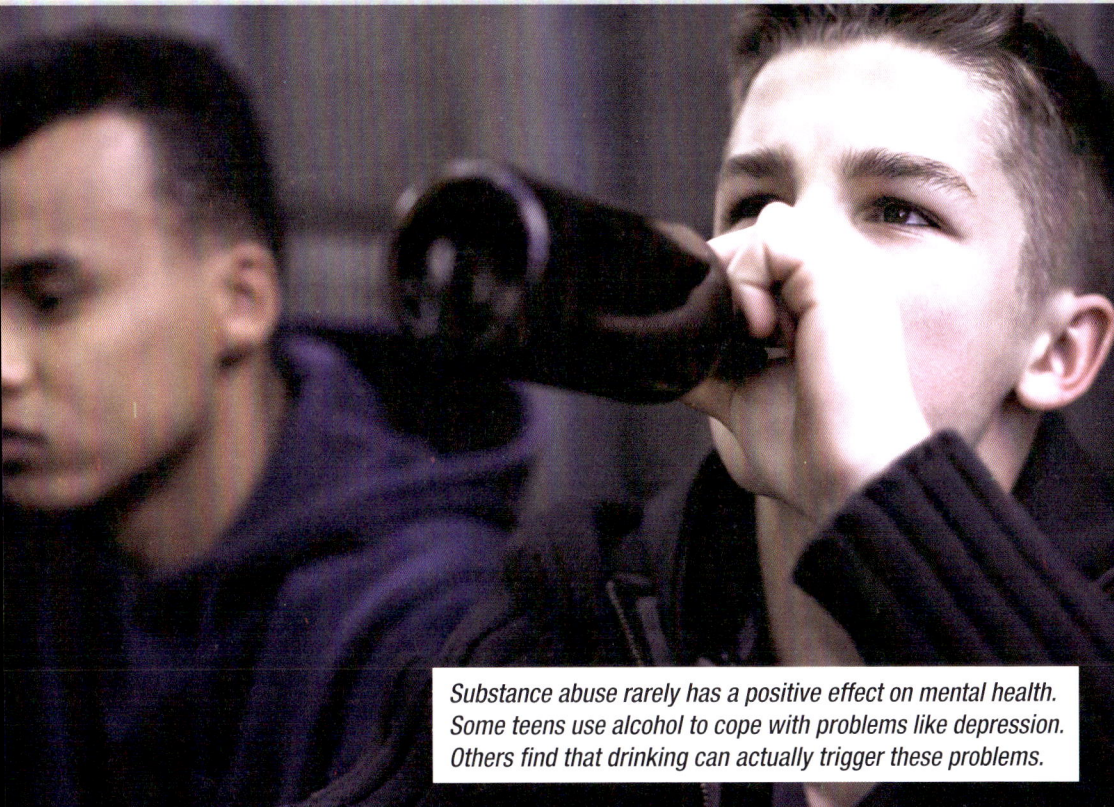

Substance abuse rarely has a positive effect on mental health. Some teens use alcohol to cope with problems like depression. Others find that drinking can actually trigger these problems.

a parent, counselor, or teacher about ways you may be able to reframe your thinking or how to find activities or classes that may be more engaging for you.

Still other mental health influences rarely have any positive benefits; substance abuse falls into this category. Some people use alcohol, marijuana, or other illegal or prescription drugs to cope with disappointment, boredom, depression, loneliness, or other problems. Some actually find that recreational drug use or drinking can trigger the onset of depression or anxiety. An estimated one in three people with a major depressive disorder also has a substance use disorder, according to American Addiction Centers.

Finally, your family's mental health history plays a large role in your experience with mental health issues, since many disorders are inheritable. Having a parent with depression, bipolar disorder, or another mental health condition does not condemn you to also suffer from such disorders, but it does mean that you might be at a higher risk for developing one. Knowing your family's medical history can be helpful for identifying early signs of trouble. "Think of mental illness as you would any other family-linked health concern," says Cleveland Clinic psychologist Scott Bea. "Do your best to become educated about the condition and symptoms so you can be on the lookout."[19]

CHAPTER THREE

Recognizing Symptoms

A person's physical health will change countless times over the course of his or her life. People get sick, get well, and get sick again. They may experience a mild cold or flu, suffer a more serious but short-term bone break, or develop a chronic illness that requires lifelong treatment. Likewise, your mental health changes many times over, in part to adapt to life's changing circumstances. "We can think of mental health as the sum total of mental, emotional, and social resources available to meet the challenges the world throws at us," says Royce Lee, an associate professor of psychiatry and behavioral neuroscience at the University of Chicago Medical Center. "When our resources run low, we start to have symptoms or difficulties. Thus, the state of our mental health is always changing depending on the balance of resources and challenges."[20]

Mental health problems aren't always obvious, like having a fever or a sore throat. You may feel like "something's wrong" but not be able to identify what it is, let alone explain it to someone else. Many people realize they have a problem when they find themselves struggling to cope with stressors that haven't changed. Not long ago, for example, you might have been able to handle a crowded hallway at school or a mall packed with customers without giving it a thought. But now, those settings might stir up a lot of anxiety. When situations remain the same but your reactions to them change—particularly if those changes feature anxiety, sadness, worthlessness, or confusion—take note and share those feelings with others.

Changes to your actions and behaviors may also indicate that something isn't quite right. Noticeable upsets to your sleeping or eating habits can indicate disorders such as depression or anxiety. Engaging in uncharacteristically reckless behaviors or withdrawing from friends or activities you like also suggest that a psychological disorder may be present.

Other behaviors that may indicate a mental health disorder is present include increased conflict and angry words with friends, parents, and others. Low energy and unexplained headaches and other symptoms are also common, as are thoughts of self-harm or persistent thoughts and memories that are hard to shake. Higher-than-normal levels of confusion, forgetfulness, and worry may also indicate a mental health disorder.

Von Conley, a senior at Ramsey High School in New Jersey, learned about such warning signs in a special course on mental health awareness offered at the school. "When we went over all the warning signs of someone who was like, spiraling, I recognized a lot of those behaviors in myself," Conley says. "When I'm not feeling great, I tend to withdraw from everyone. In the moment I felt like I needed to do something better for myself—I needed to confide in the people I love instead of hiding it."[21]

While you might experience any of these symptoms once in a while, it is a concern if they persist day after day. "While occasional bad moods and acting out can be normal adolescent conduct, these types of behaviors also can indicate underlying depression or anxiety,"[22] explains pediatrician Gurinder Dabhia.

Depression Symptoms

Depression is perplexing condition, because someone with depression can often appear to be happy and in control. Inside, however, the person may feel hopeless or even hate him- or herself. On the other hand, a person may look sad while grieving the death of a grandparent or feeling badly about not getting into the college of his or her choice. But this sadness will usually pass, and if it does, it does not constitute a depressive disorder. Depression tends to linger for long periods; if symptoms last for more than two weeks, they could indicate clinical depression.

Some of the more common symptoms of depression are those you might expect, such as persistent sadness, feelings of hopelessness, and thoughts of harming yourself or others. Withdrawing from friends, family members, and activities you once enjoyed can also suggest the onset of depression. But other feelings and behaviors are also common signs of depression, even if they may not seem so at first. If you are especially restless or irritable or have a lot of trouble concentrating, you may have depression, although those symptoms can indicate conditions such as anxiety

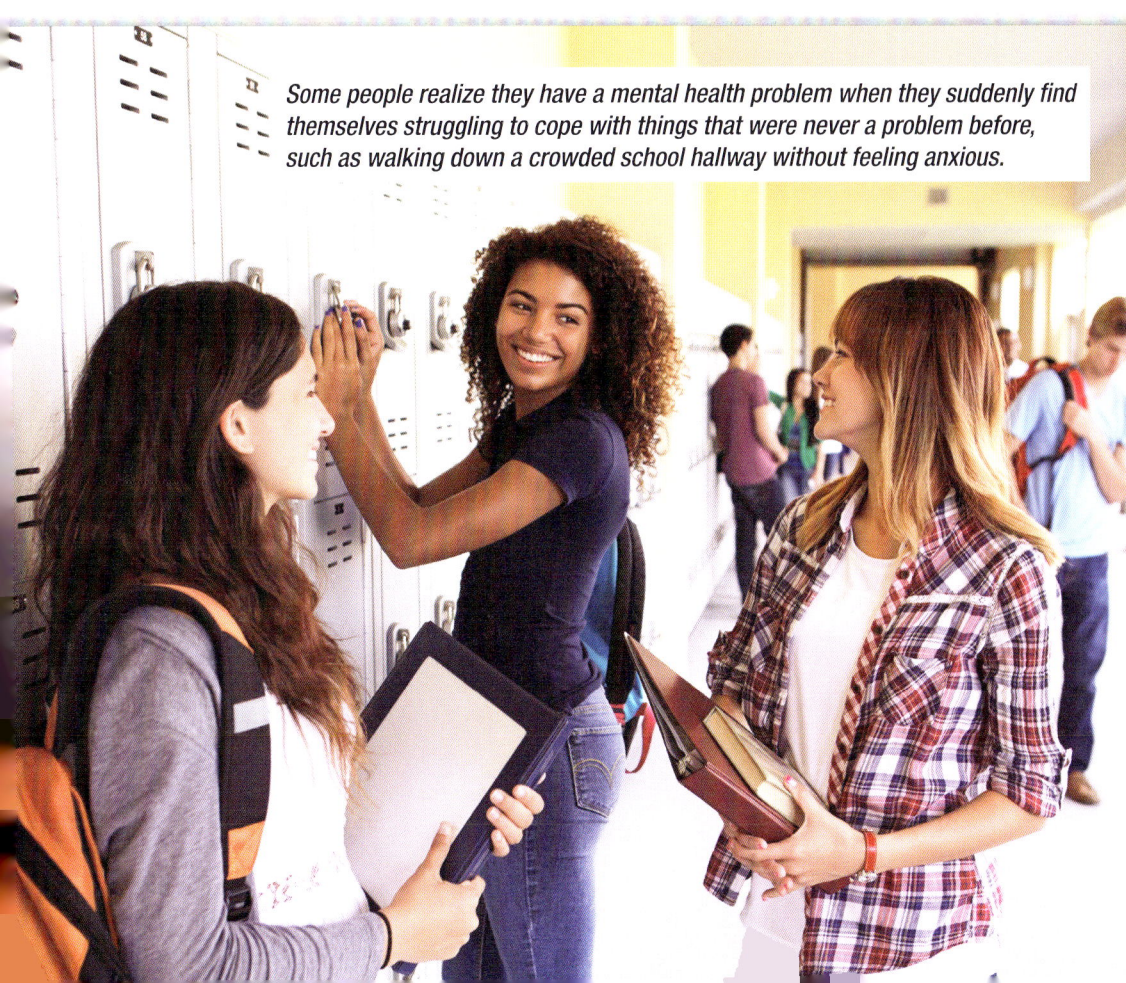

Some people realize they have a mental health problem when they suddenly find themselves struggling to cope with things that were never a problem before, such as walking down a crowded school hallway without feeling anxious.

Is It Stress or Anxiety?

Stress and anxiety share some common symptoms, like excessive worry, tension, and physical changes like high blood pressure, headaches, and sleep problems. But stress and anxiety differ in some ways, and understanding those differences can help you determine whether you are experiencing one or the other.

Stress is usually a response to an external threat or problem. Trying to finish a project on time or hearing your parents argue can trigger a lot of stress. Usually, though, stress fades once the circumstances change. Anxiety, however, is more of an internal reaction to stress, and it tends to persist, often without any specific threat or difficulty present. Another key difference is that anxiety is usually unpleasant and interferes with daily living. Stress can actually be a positive force. Going on a first date or skiing for the first time can be stressful, but they can be exciting in a positive way, too. If you're unsure whether you're experiencing prolonged stress or the possible onset of an anxiety disorder, talk about it with a parent or guardian, your doctor, a school counselor, or even a therapist if possible. Often, greater insight comes from exploring your thoughts and feelings with someone you trust.

or even attention-deficit/hyperactivity disorder. Changes in your energy level, sleeping patterns, and eating habits may be signs that you or others close to you notice, too. Changes in academic performance and school attendance can be red flags for students beginning to grapple with depression.

Alyssah Yater, a straight-A student at Killingly High School in Connecticut, developed depression and soon found herself struggling in school and experiencing other symptoms. She was one of several students to reach out to her local school board to advocate for a mental health center at her school. "You're worrying about yourself, and you're worrying about everyone else who's also struggling and trying to get them to come to school and graduate and just get through the year,"[23] Yater said in a 2022 article in the *Connecticut Mirror*.

Not everyone with depression experiences all of these symptoms. Some people may have a few, while others have many. The severity and frequency of symptoms also can vary significantly from one person to the next. Someone with major depression may also be more likely to experience multiple and more severe symptoms compared with a person who has mild depression. But even if you have just a few symptoms, you may benefit from therapy.

Anxiety Symptoms

The feelings and behaviors associated with anxiety can also vary from person to person. Some symptoms common to the nearly one-third of US adolescents estimated to have an anxiety disorder include excessive or poorly controlled worry, which is sometimes experienced as feelings of impending doom. If you have anxiety, you may also feel especially self-conscious, as though you are being judged by others. You might have trouble falling or staying asleep and feel restless and distracted much of the time. Headaches, stomachaches, and other pains may develop, too. A panic disorder or social anxiety disorder may also cause someone to experience episodes that feature a pounding or racing heart, sweating, blushing, or trembling. These disorders, as well as phobia-based disorders, may also cause a person to actively avoid situations that feel threatening. While being nervous or cautious is entirely appropriate and logical in some situations, such behavior qualifies as disordered when the level of worry doesn't match the perceived threat or if worry persists even without an obvious trigger. "The difference between normal anxiety and an actual anxiety disorder involves severity," says Cleveland Clinic psychologist Amy Lee. "Having fears and worrying is a natural reaction to stressful or new situations for children, but it's when the anxiety grows out of proportion that it becomes a real problem."[24]

PTSD Symptoms

PTSD is often associated with veterans who have been traumatized by their wartime experiences or with victims of assault. But any significant event that causes a person emotional or physical distress can lead to PTSD.

Some of the main characteristics of PTSD include intrusive memories, in which you relive a traumatic event, have nightmares related to the event, or experience distress when reminded of the event. PTSD also features negative thought and mood changes, such as increased levels of hopelessness, trouble maintaining close relationships, feeling detached from others, having memory or concentration problems, and feeling emotionally numb.

Behavior changes associated with PTSD include avoidance, which means changing the subject when the event or something similar comes up in conversation or avoiding the place, activity, or people that remind you of the event. You may also experience changes in your physical or emotional reactions, such as being easily startled, always feeling defensive or threatened, having trouble sleeping, or engaging in reckless or dangerous behaviors.

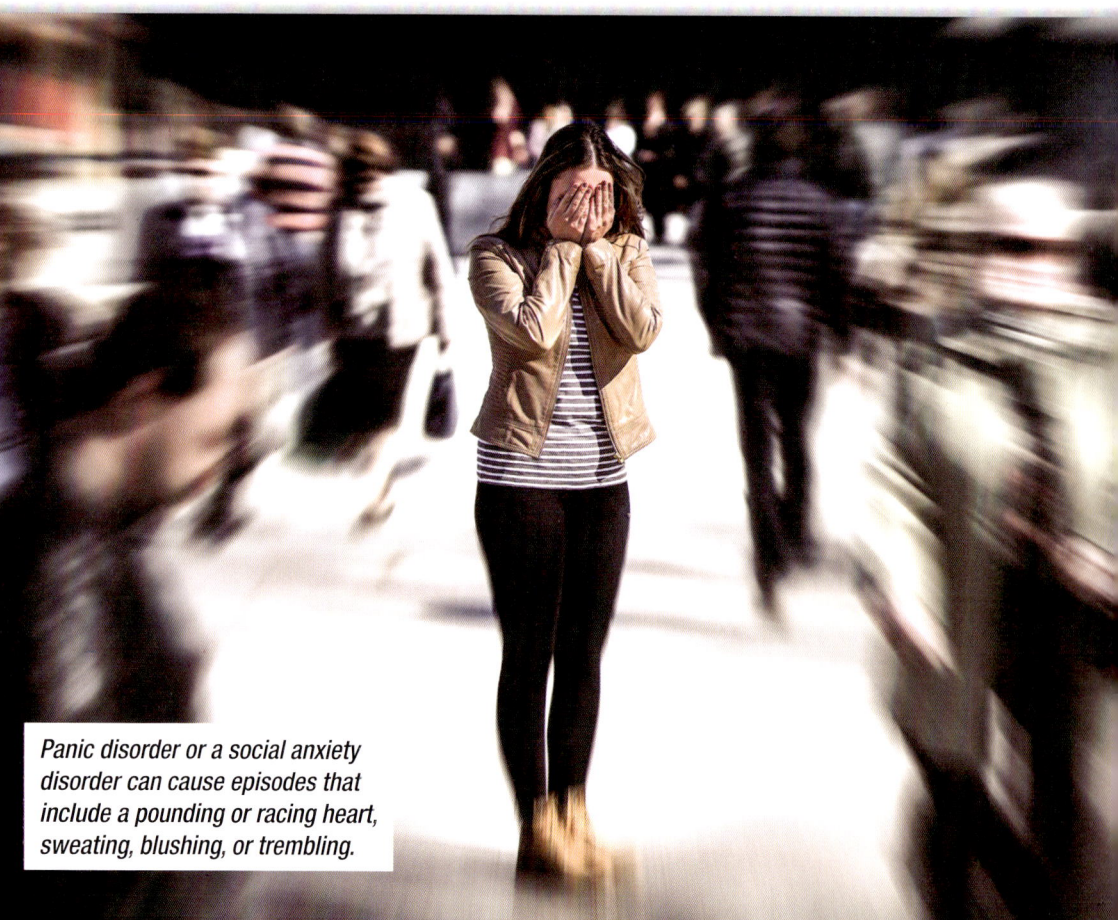

Panic disorder or a social anxiety disorder can cause episodes that include a pounding or racing heart, sweating, blushing, or trembling.

Mental Illness vs. Developmental Disorders

Even though they share some symptoms, mental illnesses are different from developmental disorders such as autism spectrum disorder, attention-deficit/hyperactivity disorder, or Down syndrome. While mental illness does not typically interfere with a person's thinking skills and memory (though it can in severe cases, especially in older adults), a developmental disorder can affect a person's ability to learn, communicate, and perform at a high level in school or work. In addition, a developmental disorder is a lifelong condition, unlike a mental illness, which can often be treated. It is also important to remember that neither mental illness nor developmental disorders are character flaws or personality defects. They can happen to anyone and are legitimate medical conditions that can be diagnosed and managed or treated, in the same way that a physical illness or injury can be diagnosed and treated.

Moods vs. Mood Disorders

Distinguishing between "normal" and "abnormal" emotions or reactions isn't always easy. Being sad, irritable, impatient, confused, frightened, angry, or otherwise upset can be a temporary or even appropriate response to an event or situation. But these feelings can also be signs of a mood disorder. As a result, teens with real mood disorders are often dismissed as simply being filled with teen angst.

Some key factors highlight the difference between a mood and a mood disorder. Happiness, for example, is an emotional state. Its opposite is sadness. Happiness and sadness are emotional states that come and go and are subject to many internal and external factors. You may experience happiness when you are cast in the lead of the school play or sadness when a friend moves away.

Depression, however, is a medical condition. It has no simple opposite, like sadness and happiness or worry and confidence. Some people may think the opposite of depression is simply happiness, but it isn't, because sadness, when experienced appropriately, is a normal human emotion. In his 2001 National Book

Award–winning memoir *The Noonday Demon: An Atlas of Depression*, author Andrew Solomon suggests that the opposite of depression might be vitality, a feeling of being alive and having energy, hope, and purpose.

Depression and sadness differ in other important ways. While you may be able to pinpoint a reason you feel sad, depression is an ongoing condition that is usually not linked to anything in particular. This is one reason why it can be hard for someone with depression to explain when someone asks, "What's wrong?"

Just as sadness and depression are often confused with each other, so too are anxiety and worry. It is natural to worry about the important people in your life and the events and situations that affect you. If a loved one is having surgery, for example, it is appropriate to worry and hope for the best. But this type of worry should ease when its cause is resolved. Everyday worries shouldn't interfere with your ability to do your homework, participate in activities, or take care of your responsibilities.

Anxiety, however, is the kind of worry that interferes with your ability to enjoy yourself, get your work done, get a good night's sleep, and otherwise carry out your normal functions and experience peaceful moments. For Nashua (New Hampshire) North High School student Mia Flegal, the earliest symptom of her generalized anxiety disorder was an awful feeling in her belly. "That pit in your stomach starts to creep its way up to your chest, and it feels like someone is compressing you," she said in a Seacoastonline.com article in 2022. She'd wake up in a cold sweat and sometimes feel like she couldn't breathe. "You didn't see an end to it, and it's so hard."[25] Eventually, Flegal reached out for help and realized that talking about anxiety with others was the first step toward regaining control.

If these challenges are present in your life, tell a parent, doctor, or someone you trust. Responding promptly to any type of symptom is always the smart approach.

Self-Harm and Suicidal Thoughts

The ways people react to emotional pain can vary dramatically, from avoidance and denial to committing acts of self-harm and

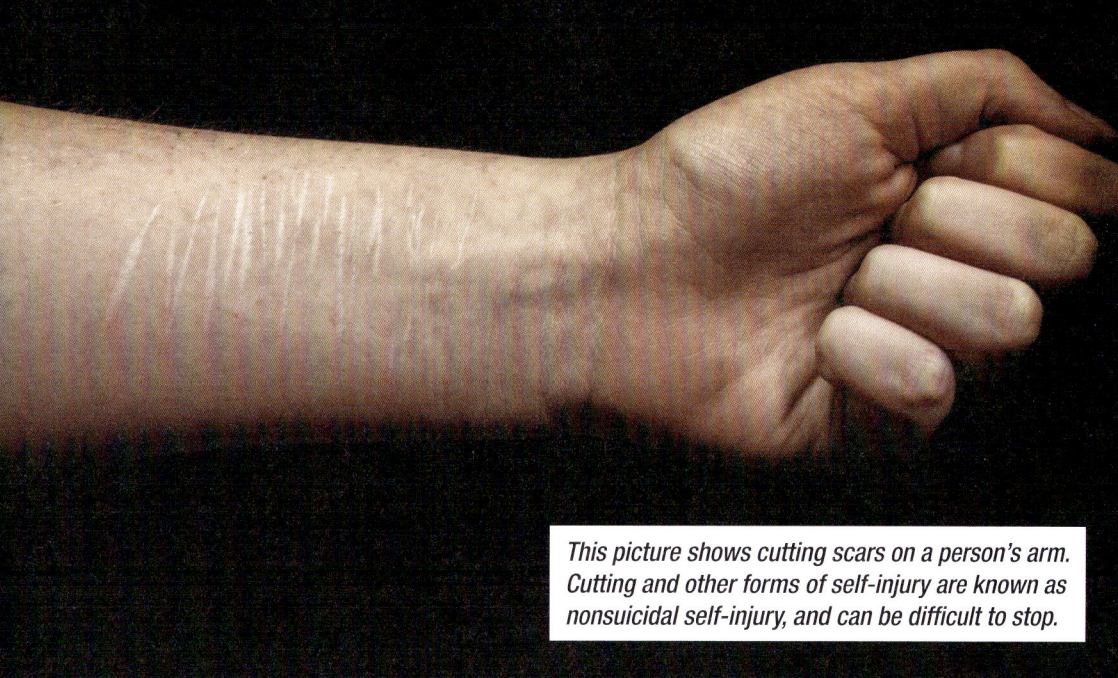

This picture shows cutting scars on a person's arm. Cutting and other forms of self-injury are known as nonsuicidal self-injury, and can be difficult to stop.

thinking about suicide. No matter their source, such thoughts and behaviors are signs that help is needed immediately.

Cutting, head banging, hair pulling, scratching until the skin bleeds, and other forms of self-injury are known as nonsuicidal self-injury (NSSI). While engaging in NSSI may not represent a desire to die, research suggests that teens who have trouble stopping NSSI could face higher risks of experiencing suicidal thoughts or attempting suicide compared with their peers in the general public.

If you notice that a friend has scars or other signs of cutting or NSSI, consider asking about it in a kind, nonjudgmental, or noncritical way. Be willing to listen. Encourage your friend to talk with a trusted adult; you could offer to go with your friend to the conversation. If your friend doesn't want to talk about it, which is common, tell a trusted adult about your concerns.

If a friend discusses suicide, even in an offhanded manner, tell an adult immediately. And if you have such thoughts, talk with your parents, teachers, doctor, or anyone you trust who will listen. And remember that treatment for that pain is possible, and whatever you are going through can be managed.

It may also help to know that many other young people are struggling, too. A 2023 survey by the Centers for Disease Control and Prevention (CDC) showed that 60 percent of teenage girls in the United States reported feeling sadness every day for at least two weeks in the previous year and that one in three teen girls had considered suicide. These statistics followed a 2020 CDC report that found that more than 13 percent of US kids ages three to seventeen had a current diagnosed mental health or behavioral condition. This represented an increase of 60 percent from 2007. "Mental health challenges in children, adolescents and young adults are real and they are widespread," said US surgeon general Vivek Murthy in 2022. "Even before the pandemic, an alarming number of young people struggled with feelings of helplessness, depression and thoughts of suicide— and rates have increased over the past decade."[26]

Don't Ignore Your Feelings

Even if you are knowledgeable about the symptoms and signs associated with mental illness, you may find yourself having thoughts or feelings that don't seem to fit neatly into a particular category. That's okay and is a fairly universal experience. Most people have days or weeks when they just don't feel right or like themselves. Allow yourself to feel how you feel without shame or self-consciousness. Don't assume the worst, but listen to your gut. If something doesn't feel right, respect that sensation rather than ignore it or downplay it. If uneasiness persists, share your thoughts and feelings with someone else, even if you can't really describe them clearly. Just talking about them may help.

CHAPTER FOUR

Self-Care Strategies

Staying in good physical health means eating a balanced diet, getting regular exercise, and avoiding injury and illness. If you do get sick or hurt, it is important to see a doctor, take appropriate medication, receive treatment, and simply rest.

The same is true for managing your mental health. In addition to living a physically healthy lifestyle, it is important to learn stress-management techniques and to practice self-care. Managing your mental health also means dealing with ongoing challenges, as well as unexpected crises, with positive and constructive responses. Taking care of body and mind gives you the best chance of maintaining your well-being.

Exercise

The mood-boosting benefits of exercise are well established. Numerous studies have found a strong link between regular physical activity and reduced symptoms of stress, anxiety, and depression. You don't need to work out for hours a day to achieve a benefit. "Even just walking just three times a week seems to give people better mental health than not exercising at all,"[27] says psychiatry professor Adam Chekroud, coauthor of a 2018 mental health study involving more than 1.2 million people.

Exercise supports mental health in several ways. Physical activity triggers the release of endorphins and other brain chemicals that support a brighter mood and better sense of well-being. At the same time, exercise reduces levels of stress hormones, such as cortisol and adrenaline. Exercise—especially aerobic activity that gives your lungs and heart a

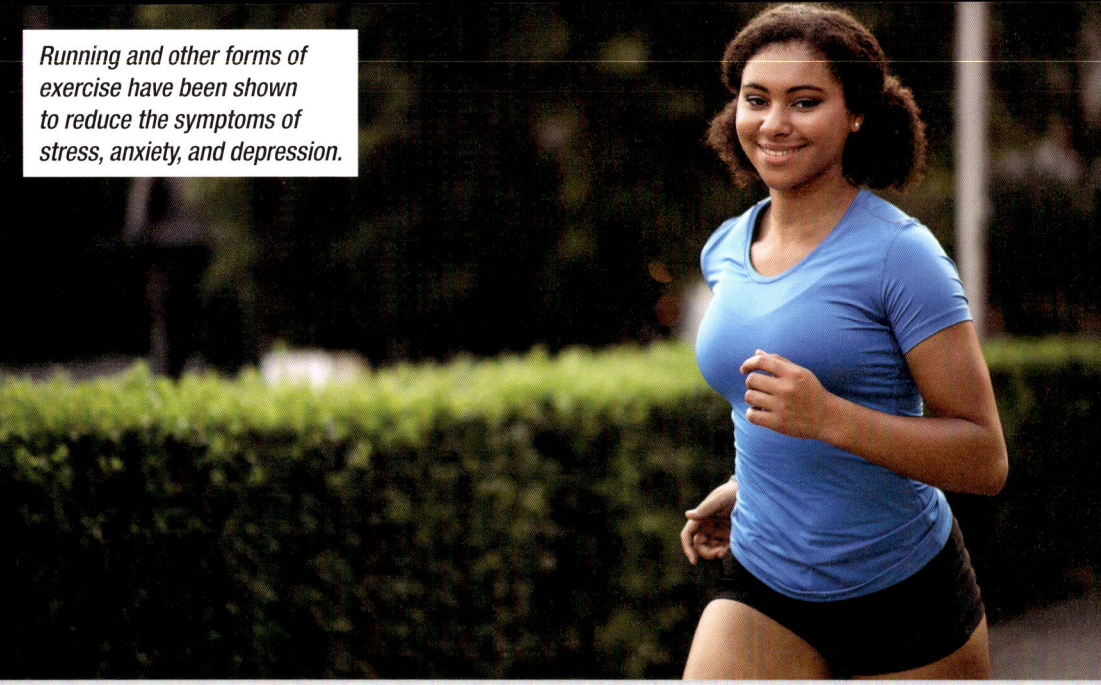

Running and other forms of exercise have been shown to reduce the symptoms of stress, anxiety, and depression.

workout—improves circulation to the brain, which supports better emotional regulation and thinking skills.

Meeting exercise and fitness goals can also improve your confidence and self-esteem. Exercise that features group or team sports also serves your mental health because it has a social component to it.

Taking a walk, playing sports, dancing, and doing other physical activities can help take your mind off your problems, which in turn can help you relax and even find a new perspective on things. In a 2021 essay in *Psychology Today*, psychologist Kenneth E. Miller wrote that when you go for a walk or run or take a similar break from trying to solve a difficult problem, your unconscious mind keeps working on it, while your conscious mind has left it behind. "By shifting our attention away from the problem that's vexing us, we quiet the mind and turn down the volume on our thinking," he says. "That opens up a space to listen more closely to what we are feeling, to hear our own inner wisdom."[28]

An Australian study published in 2023 found that regular exercise could be even more helpful than medications for certain people dealing with mental health disorders. Lead researcher Ben Singh explains that short workouts of higher intensity exercise had greater improvements for depression and anxiety, while longer durations had smaller effects when compared to short and mid-duration bursts. We also found that all types of physical activity and exercise were beneficial, including aerobic exercise such as walking, resistance training, Pilates, and yoga. Importantly, the research shows that it doesn't take much for exercise to make a positive change to your mental health.[29]

Eat a Healthy Diet

An eating strategy that emphasizes fruits, vegetables, whole grains, lean proteins, and other sources of important nutrients will support good mental health better than a diet packed with processed foods, empty calories, and junk food. A 2022 study in the journal *Public Health Nutrition* found that people who ate the most ultraprocessed food (soda, chips, french fries, candy, etc.) were more likely to report symptoms of mild depression and have more anxious days per month.

It is also healthy to eat at least one meal a day with a family member. Conflicting work schedules, school, and extracurricular activities can make this difficult, but the benefits can be substantial, explains pediatrician Channing Brown. "Eating one meal a day as a family is associated with a decreased risk of certain mental health conditions, such as depression, poor academic performance, and substance abuse, and is specifically protective against eating disorders in children and teenagers,"[30] says Brown.

> "Eating one meal a day as a family is associated with a decreased risk of certain mental health conditions, such as depression, poor academic performance, and substance abuse."[30]
>
> —Channing Brown, pediatrician

Get Enough Sleep

Getting enough sleep is the third and perhaps most underrated aspect of mental and physical health. Every year, new research underscores how good sleep helps lower the risk of mood disorders

The Power of Journaling

Journals serve many purposes throughout your life. They can offer records of and observations about daily events. They can hold your dreams, goals, and ideas. And when it comes to mental health, journals can be especially helpful. Your mental health depends on your ability to express yourself in a healthy way. You can practice this skill by writing down your problems, fears, and feelings, knowing they won't be judged or misunderstood, because a journal is private. Sometimes in therapy, it can be helpful to share journal passages because they represent a "real-time" record of how you were feeling at a particular moment. But even if you keep your journal just for you, it can help you recognize triggers or strategies that help you cope. You can also fill your journal with positive self-talk.

A journal doesn't have to be an expensive leather-bound book. A simple spiral notebook can do the job. To make it effective, try to write for at least a few minutes every day, and don't worry about grammar and punctuation. Just know that you're helping yourself however and whatever you write.

and how poor sleep leads to a decline in thinking skills and reduced immunity to infection and illness. A 2022 British study, for example, found that teens who suffered from insomnia or had late bedtimes on school nights were much more likely to experience emotional and behavioral struggles than their peers who had earlier bedtimes and sufficient sleep.

The Centers for Disease Control and Prevention advises that teens ages thirteen to eighteen get eight to ten hours of sleep per twenty-four hours. Those hours should be uninterrupted and in the 10:00 p.m. to 7:00 a.m. range. Even though sleeping from 2:00 a.m. to 7:00 a.m. and 3:00 p.m. to 6:00 p.m. totals eight hours, your body and mind will benefit much more from an uninterrupted eight hours of nighttime sleep. "The time of night when you sleep makes a significant difference in terms of the structure and quality of your sleep,"[31] says Matt Walker, head of the Sleep and Neuroimaging Lab at the University of California, Berkeley.

Socialize

Regularly interacting with others is an essential part of optimal mental health at any age. The key is to engage with others who bring positivity into your life. Try to maintain a social network of at least a few friends who provide emotional support, inspiration, laughter, and other valuable qualities.

Having regular contact with friends means you're surrounding yourself with people who will boost your self-esteem, listen to your problems, and remind you of your connection and importance to the world around you. "Friends can improve your self-confidence and self-worth," says Mahzad Hojjat, a psychology professor at the University of Massachusetts, Dartmouth. "You want to have friends to share in your success who are happy for you."[32]

Manage Your Stress

Learning to manage stress is one of the most important skills for maintaining your mental health and lowering your risk of emotional

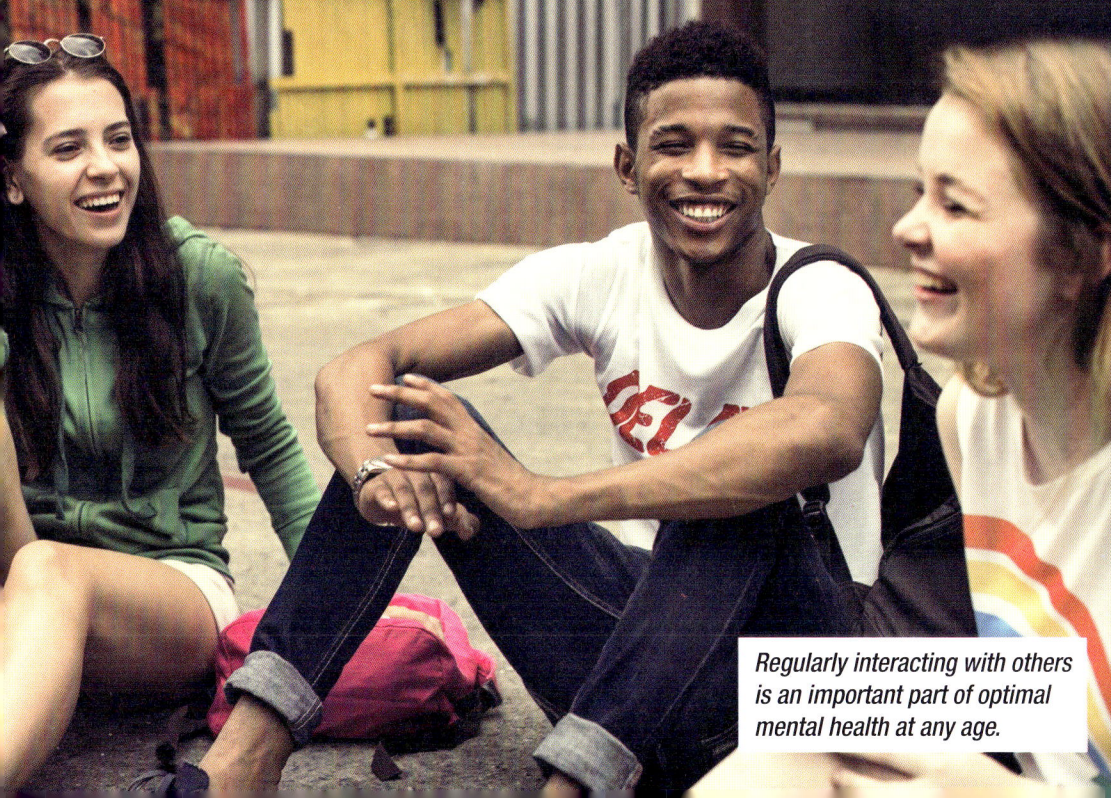

Regularly interacting with others is an important part of optimal mental health at any age.

Listen to the People You Trust

If your parents, friends, or siblings continuously ask you questions like "Is everything okay?" and "What's wrong?" or start pointing out changes they're noticing, you may be inclined to get defensive or deny that anything is wrong. It is natural to want to keep uncomfortable feelings to yourself. But make an effort to hear your friends and family out. The people who know you best are often the first ones to notice changes that may be signs of heightened stress or a mental health disorder. They may point out unusual behaviors or statements that are deeply concerning but that you may not have noticed or been aware of at the time. And just as importantly, friends and loved ones may be able to offer truly helpful advice and perspectives that may get you through a difficult time. When people you trust express concern or offer to help, take them at their word. Likewise, think twice about taking the advice or following the lead of someone you don't trust or respect. Ask yourself if this person really has your best interests at heart. If not, look elsewhere for support and guidance.

and psychological problems later on. Kim Goodman, a behavioral health specialist and professor in the University of Southern California's School of Social Work, notes that poorly controlled stress can lead to long-term mental health disorders, as well as reckless or dangerous behaviors in the short term. "Chronic stress can lead to depression, anxiety, low tolerance levels and interpersonal relationship challenges,"[33] Goodman says, adding that stress can also lead people to try managing it with alcohol, drugs, or other high-risk choices.

Whether it's meditation, yoga, deep-breathing techniques or other strategies, what's most important is to find an approach that works for you and is something you will do regularly. Maybe taking your dog for a walk helps you relax. Maybe shooting hoops in the gym centers you. Maybe you feel calm when you watch silly cat videos or cooking shows. Find a healthy stress reliever that works for you, and prioritize it. Schedule stress-relief time into your day the same way you do homework, chores, or other obligations.

Another key part of stress management is to follow age-old advice that goes something like "Focus only on what you can control, and learn to accept that you can't control everything." Of course, this is much easier said than done. It can be helpful to identify which aspects of life are under your control. What you eat, how much you study, and how you respond to various situations are all your choices.

Be Your Own Best Friend

Think about how you would talk to a friend who was feeling confused, sad, worried, or overwhelmed. You would probably be supportive and kind and offer helpful advice. Take that same approach with yourself. "Positive self-talk is one of the most valuable tools you can use to keep yourself emotionally and mentally balanced,"[34] says therapist Barton Goldsmith.

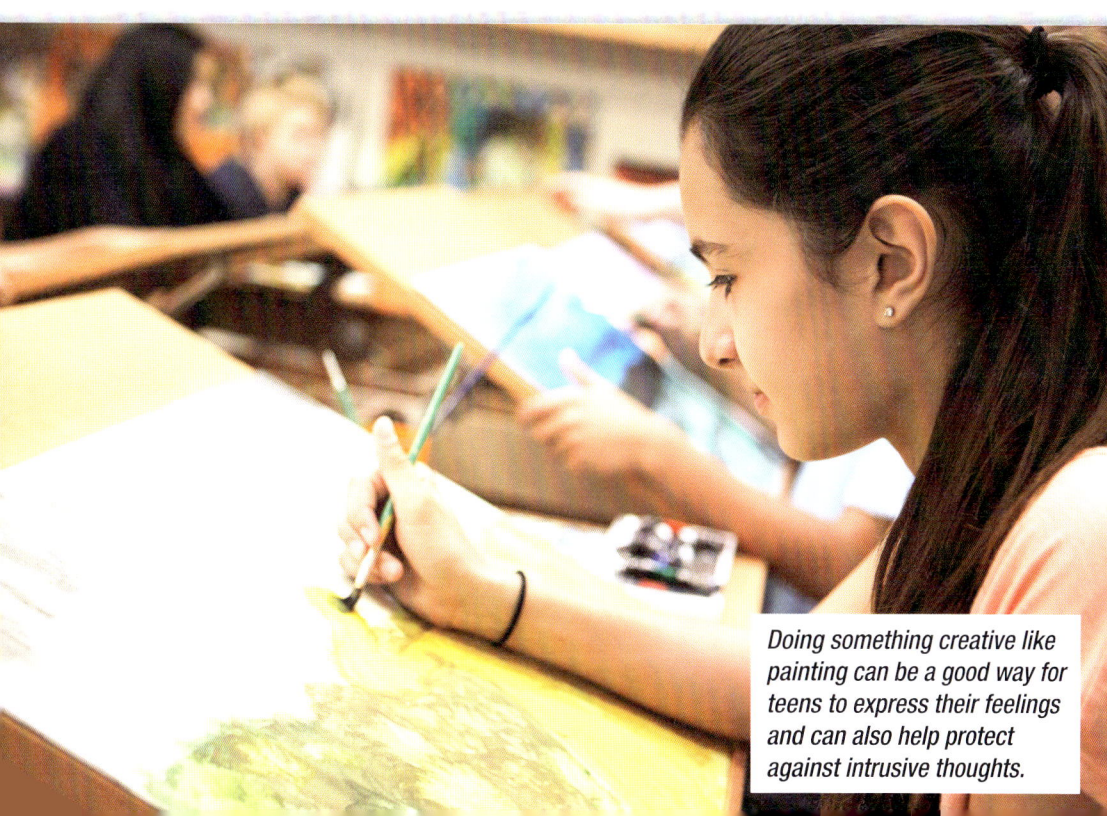

Doing something creative like painting can be a good way for teens to express their feelings and can also help protect against intrusive thoughts.

Think about your strengths and successes. Just as you might brainstorm solutions or new approaches to a friend's vexing problems, do the same for yourself. Remember that you are resourceful and resilient and have survived to this point, so think about how you can make the next chapter or even just the next day better, more productive, or more manageable than the day before.

Other Self-Care Strategies

As you look for ways to de-stress and take care of yourself, consider volunteering, which helps you get out of your own head for a bit. Research also suggests that the feel-good brain chemicals that are released when we give to others are more rewarding than when we receive a gift.

Also consider setting down your phone and giving yourself a break from social media, the news, or any other screen-based stimuli. This worked for a group of teens who live in Brooklyn, New York, who formed an anti-technology group they called the Luddite Club. Club members got rid of their smartphones and swapped them for flip phones, which don't connect to apps like Instagram or Snapchat. The teens said getting off of social media was a relief and opened them up to appreciating simpler things. "The best part about being a Luddite is my self-awareness," Biruk Watling told Chalkbeat New York, a nonprofit online news organization that covers education. "I have time to reflect about my day and my life."[35]

You can always try doing something creative, like writing, drawing, dancing, or making music to ease your stress. Take an arts class. Creative expression helps you express your feelings and may help protect against intrusive thoughts. Even reading or listening to music—appreciating the creative expression of others—is associated with lower levels of loneliness, because it connects you to the thoughts and ideas of others.

CHAPTER FIVE

Reaching Out for Help

If you are struggling with your mental health, it may be time to see a mental health professional. You may not need ongoing therapy; checking in periodically with a counselor might be enough to help you handle stress or deal with problems. Conversely, you may benefit from regular, weekly therapy sessions to treat a diagnosed mental health disorder or other challenge.

You don't need a diagnosis to benefit from therapy. Mental health services can help people struggling with relationship problems, gender identity, and stress management. "We all experience issues at some point in our lives, whether it be a bad breakup, a stressful work situation, or family difficulties," says licensed clinical social worker Sal Raichbach. "Talking to someone who is trained in handling emotions and working out problems can be extremely beneficial."[36]

Most important to know is that you don't have to go through any crisis alone. Somebody, somewhere will take the time to listen. Just don't ignore your symptoms or put off getting help. The US Department of Health and Human Services reports that only about half of the children and teens with diagnosable mental health conditions get the treatment they need.

The first person you open up to might be a family member, friend, teacher, school counselor, or family doctor. Lacey McPhee, a high school junior from La Crosse, Wisconsin, says that opening up to her parents made her challenges more manageable. "I've had mental health illnesses and struggles, and I taught my mom and my dad a little bit on the best way to be there for me," she told Governor Tony Evers in a 2021 state roundtable on children's mental health awareness. "And so over the years, it's definitely been so much better, and my mom is like my biggest support system."[37]

Getting help early gives you the best chance of having positive outcomes. This is because the developing brain can be more responsive to treatment compared with the brain of an older adult. As you approach adulthood, your brain is forming grooves and ridges to expand its surface area to make room for more brain cells involved in thinking, emotions, motor skills, and other functions. "Once you have a diagnosis, act quickly, when psychotherapy or medications are most effective," says Cleveland Clinic psychologist Scott Bea. "If you allow habits to develop, the brain circuits and grooves deepen, and it becomes more challenging to overcome."[38]

Getting a Mental Health Evaluation

If you feel a cold coming on, you probably don't rush to the doctor. But if your symptoms get worse or don't go away, you will likely seek out care. Seeing a mental health professional isn't that different. Early, mild feelings of restlessness, sadness, or worry might be manageable or chalked up to a stressful week. Worsening symptoms, however, warrant a visit to a counselor or other mental health professional.

At your first visit, expect to answer all kinds of questions about your daily life and routine; sleep and diet behaviors; family environment; history of trauma; school challenges and successes; relationships, including with friends and romantic partners; social skills; mood swings; psychological functioning; and more. These details are intended to give the therapist information and insight into your life: The more you share, the more effective the sessions will be. "It's OK to be nervous!" says psychologist Gina Delucca. "You're meeting someone for the first time who is likely going to ask you some very personal and emotionally sensitive questions and you're expected to be very honest and forthcoming with them. It's a very unnatural and nerve-inducing type of situation, and as therapists we try to be sensitive to this."[39]

If a diagnosable mental health disorder is suspected, you will want an accurate diagnosis. Receiving a diagnosis gives you a name and a definition for your condition. The right diagnosis also determines appropriate treatment options and allows health insurance providers to determine what treatments should be covered. To receive a proper diagnosis, you will undergo a physical examination to rule out any physical reasons for your symptoms, as well as lab tests to check for things like thyroid function, which can affect mood. You will also have a psychological evaluation, which includes a careful review of symptoms.

Mental health disorder symptoms are listed in the *Diagnostic and Statistical Manual of Mental Disorders* (DSM), published by the American Psychiatric Association, which updates the manual

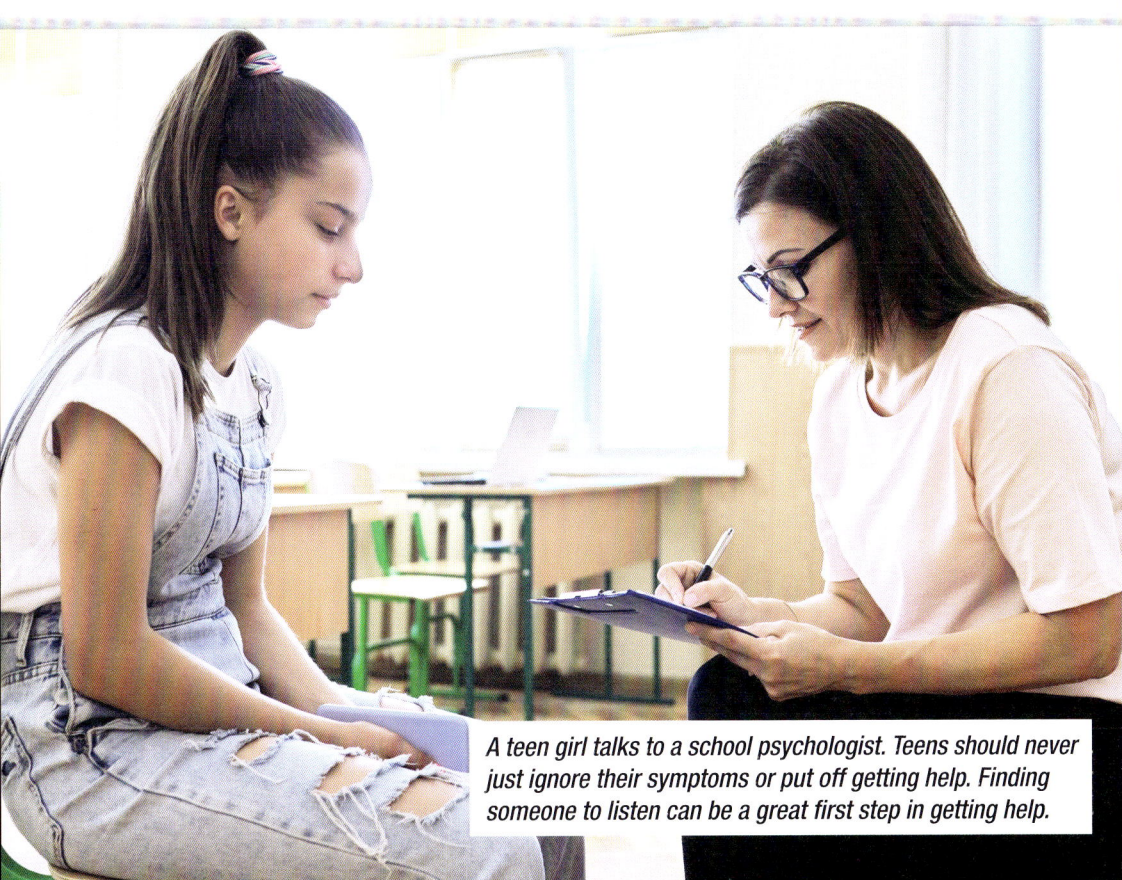

A teen girl talks to a school psychologist. Teens should never just ignore their symptoms or put off getting help. Finding someone to listen can be a great first step in getting help.

periodically to keep up with current research. For example, some of the criteria listed for a formal diagnosis of depression include "depressed mood most of the day, nearly every day," and a "markedly diminished interest or pleasure in all, or almost all, activities most of the day, nearly every day."[40]

A person typically needs to meet certain criteria listed in the DSM for that disorder to be officially diagnosed. If your symptoms don't result in a specific diagnosis, your therapist may say you tend toward a particular disorder and may suggest treatment that includes healthier lifestyle adjustments (getting more sleep and exercise, for example) or ongoing talk therapy. If therapy is the plan, then you need to approach it as a partnership between you and your therapist, both working toward an agreed-upon goal.

Goals of Therapy

At the outset of therapy, the client (patient) and therapist develop a set of goals based on the person's needs and desires. The goals are arrived at mutually after a few conversations and should be ambitious but realistic. For example, you might want a healthier relationship with your parents. Family therapy might help all of you learn to communicate calmly and more effectively and understand each other's point of view more clearly. But it would be unrealistic to expect that you and your parents will never disagree about anything again. With therapy, however, those disagreements may be handled with more kindness and understanding in the future.

Once goals are established, the next step is to determine whether therapy is actually helping. "When I work with clients, I like to have them articulate their goals, and we put them in writing together," says psychologist Ruth Varkovitzky. "We also try to identify how we would know if things were getting better, and how we want to measure progress."[41] Sometimes the ideas and

> "When I work with clients, I like to have them articulate their goals, and we put them in writing together. We also try to identify how we would know if things were getting better, and how we want to measure progress."[41]
>
> —Ruth Varkovitzky, psychologist

Telehealth Therapy

Getting access to mental health services isn't always easy, especially when you're young or if there are few resources available where you live. But mental health is one field in which telehealth—medical services provided via computer, phone, or video chat—can nearly duplicate the experience of in-person care. "You can do psychotherapy and mental health care very well if you have a good quality audio-visual connection," says Paul Desan, director of the Psychiatric Consultation Service at Yale New Haven Hospital. "It's much easier for people to schedule a visit and they don't have to drive there and then wait to be seen."

The COVID-19 pandemic was the main driver of mental telehealth's growth. A study from the Kaiser Family Foundation noted that only about 1 percent of mental health services were administered via video chat or phone in 2019, but by the summer of 2020, the number had jumped to 13 percent, and a year later more than one-third of outpatient mental health care was delivered through telehealth platforms. "I don't think the mental health system will ever go back to all in-person sessions," says Desan.

Quoted in Carrie MacMillan, "Why Telehealth for Mental Health Is Working," YaleMedicine, September 16, 2021. www.yalemedicine.org.

strategies discussed in therapy don't help, so you may need to try new approaches or even change therapists.

While every person who begins therapy will have unique goals particular to their circumstances, there are some common themes shared by many people in counseling. Among them are the following:

- Moving away from or replacing behaviors that are unhelpful or harmful (such as replacing drug use or other dangerous activities with martial arts or music classes.)
- Improving the ability to begin and/or maintain relationships
- Learning to cope with new or existing challenges

- Becoming more effective in school, work, or other activities
- Improving decision-making skills and using better judgment
- Improving self-confidence and self-esteem

Effective therapists create specific goals based on their patients' needs. For example, someone with an eating disorder such as anorexia nervosa would set out to change the thoughts and behaviors that are contributing to restrictive eating. If a patient struggled with being in a crowd, therapy goals would include understanding why crowds make him or her anxious and developing strategies to help the person cope in those situations. "I think of therapy like building a toolbox," says Cleveland Clinic psychologist Amy Lee. "You don't need every tool every day. But by having them, you're prepared. In therapy, we try to build resiliency by identifying gaps in the toolbox and filling them in."[42]

Types of Therapy

The right type of therapy for you depends on the nature of your mental health concerns, your comfort level with certain approaches, and the availability and affordability of therapy options in your community.

Cognitive behavioral therapy (CBT), for example, is based on the idea that if you can learn to think differently about a situation, your feelings and behaviors will then change, too. The goal is to replace unrealistic and unhelpful thoughts with realistic and constructive ones that will lead to more positive emotions and behaviors that will better serve you. For British teenager Sophie Goldstone, CBT helped her understand and manage her OCD and realize that the disorder was not a life sentence. She had experienced horrifying intrusive thoughts about her family and was unable to go into certain rooms in her house or wear certain clothes because she feared they'd been contaminated. "The first

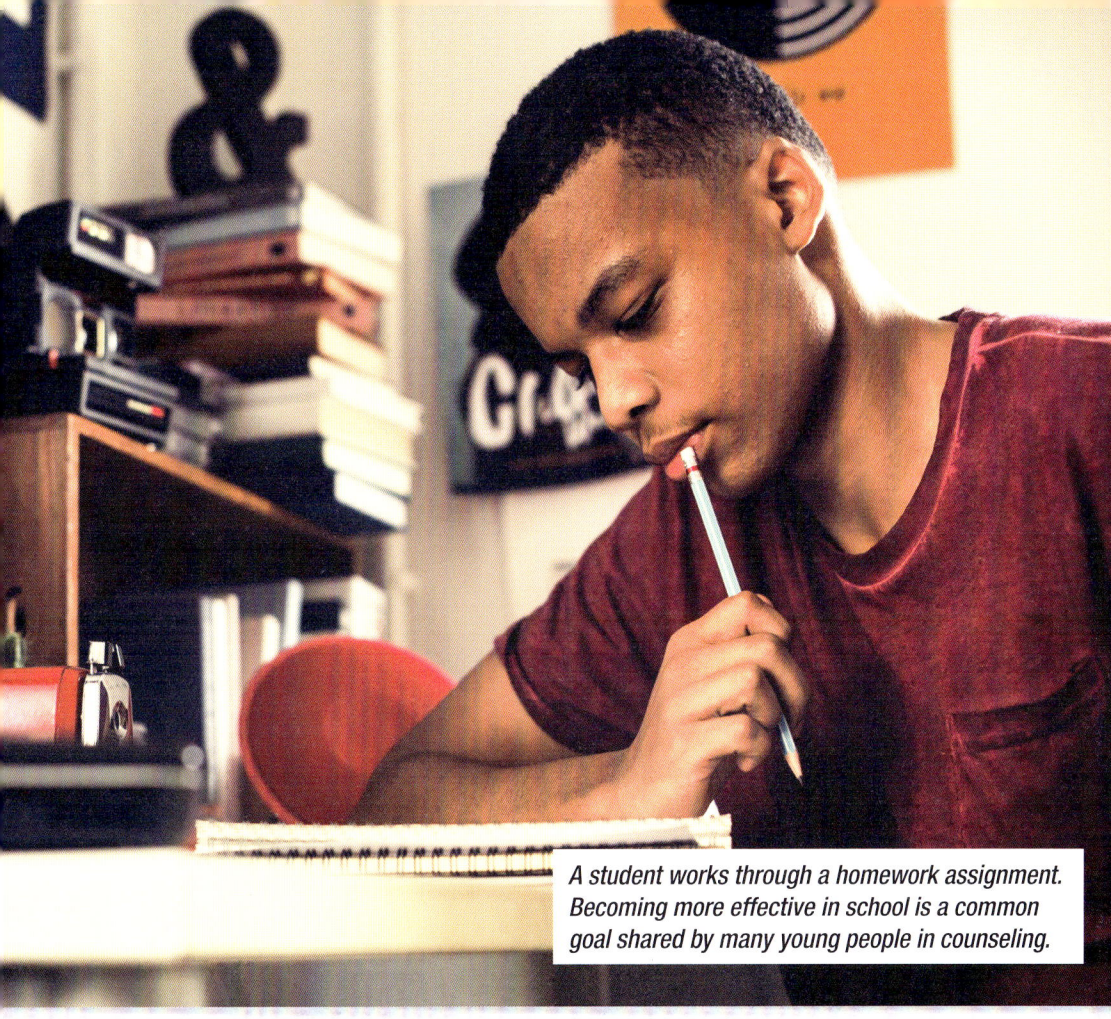

A student works through a homework assignment. Becoming more effective in school is a common goal shared by many young people in counseling.

few weeks of treatment were good," she shares. "I learned from clinical psychologists exactly what I was going through—what my OCD meant, and why. I finally started to understand it as an illness, and that I could get better. That it wasn't just me, and what I felt was treatable."[43]

There are many other types of therapy to explore. Among them are dialectical behavioral therapy, a type of CBT that is usually employed when people have extreme emotional challenges. It focuses more on changing behavior patterns rather than thinking and talking through issues. There is also family counseling, which involves parents and their kids, sometimes meeting as a group and at other times meeting individually with a therapist. It often focuses on improving communication and conflict resolution. Interpersonal therapy is a specific type of psychotherapy focused on improving a person's ability to interact with and relate to others. It is often used to help people when a breakup or the loss of a friend or family member leads to deepening levels of depression. Acceptance and commitment therapy helps a person learn to stop denying or avoiding certain feelings and emotions and accept that they are appropriate to certain situations in order to move forward in life.

A person's therapeutic needs may change with life's circumstances. For example, family therapy may be helpful for teens, but CBT may be more appropriate for people later in life. The key is to be aware of whether the treatment you are receiving seems to be helping—and if not, it is okay to switch gears and try a different kind.

Moving Forward

Maintaining your mental well-being throughout life can be an ongoing challenge. No matter your age, it is important to maintain

Types of Mental Health Professionals

Just as there are many types of physicians, there are also numerous kinds of mental health professionals. Psychiatrists are licensed to diagnose mental health disorders, treat individuals with talk therapy, and prescribe medications. A psychiatrist is a medical doctor (MD) who has graduated from medical school. Advanced practice psychiatric nurses can also prescribe medications.

Psychologists are licensed to diagnose mental health disorders and provide therapy for a range of emotional, behavioral, and psychological concerns. Psychologists hold advanced degrees but are not MDs and cannot prescribe medications.

Mental health counselors are licensed to provide individual and group therapy. Two common types of mental health counselors include licensed clinical social workers and licensed professional counselors. Other mental health professionals include pastoral counselors, who work through churches and other religious organizations, as well as therapists who focus on certain areas, such as family or couples counseling, adolescent and pediatric therapy, sports psychology, grief counseling, and many other areas.

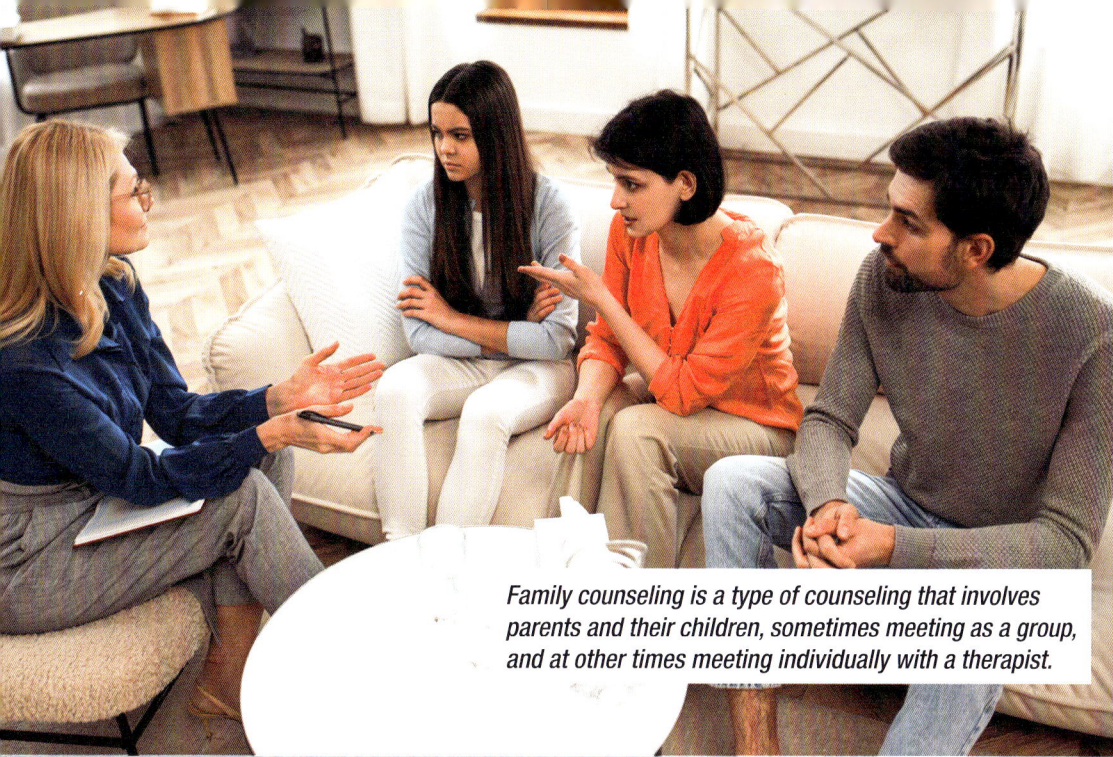

Family counseling is a type of counseling that involves parents and their children, sometimes meeting as a group, and at other times meeting individually with a therapist.

a healthy lifestyle and get professional help should you feel that your mental health is starting to suffer.

Above all, remember that good mental health is not a static, lifelong quality, like being tall or having brown eyes. Rather, your mental health is like a plant. It needs to be regularly tended to and cared for to thrive. Jen Sincore Gallagher, a psychologist, says:

> Many people are surprised by the notion that good mental health requires proactive and deliberate care. . . . Sometimes our methods of emotion management and expression that work well in one stage of our lives do not translate to the next. Sometimes our coping skills work for a while and then do not work as well later. This is true even when the circumstances do not change. This is normal.[44]

The better prepared you are to recognize good and poor mental health, the better able you are to promptly respond to life changes as they occur. And the more confidence and self-awareness you have, the more willing and able you will be to reach out for help.

SOURCE NOTES

Introduction: Your Mind and You

1. Quoted in Rose Minutaglio, "Selena Gomez and Dr. Jill Biden Sit Down to Discuss Mental Health," Yahoo! News, May 19, 2022. https://news.yahoo.com.
2. Quoted in White House, "Remarks of President Joe Biden—State of the Union Address as Prepared for Delivery," February 7, 2023. www.whitehouse.gov.
3. Quoted in Cleveland Clinic, "How to Choose the Best Child Therapy and Therapist," January 11, 2023. https://health.clevelandclinic.org.
4. Quoted in Michael Ordona, "Selena Gomez Finds Her Balance and Shares Her Struggle in the Song 'My Mind & Me,'" *Los Angeles Times*, January 10, 2023. www.latimes.com.

Chapter One: The Meaning of Mental Health

5. Quoted in Chelsea Johnson, "Defining and Understanding Mental Health," University of Chicago Medicine, May 12, 2022. www.uchicagomedicine.org.
6. Quoted in Melinda Wenner Moyer, "Teens Are Struggling Right Now. What Can Parents Do?," *New York Times*, February 20, 2023. www.nytimes.com.
7. Quoted in Vital Beat, "We All Have Mental Health," May 6, 2019. www.thevitalbeat.ca.
8. Quoted in Katia Hetter, "Anxiety Disorders Are Common. Here's What Everyone Should Know About Them," CNN, October 13, 2022. www.cnn.com.
9. Quoted in *NIH News in Health*, "Understanding Anxiety Disorders," March 2016. https://newsinhealth.nih.gov.
10. Quoted in Meg St. Espirit, "Teen Helps Start School Mental Health Club After Her Own Loss, Depression," *Pittsburgh (PA) City Paper*, January 5, 2022. www.pghcitypaper.com.
11. Quoted in Samantha Manning, "High School Student Urges Lawmakers to Help Teens Struggling with Their Mental Health," WSB-TV, December 4, 2022. www.wsbtv.com.
12. Quoted in Rebekah Hall, "CDC Study Reveals Mental Health Crisis Among High School Students; Tips for Parents," The Arkadelphian, March 16, 2023. https://arkadelphian.com.

13. Quoted in Kate Wells, "As More Teens Are Hospitalized for Eating Disorders, Here's What Parents Need to Know," Michigan Radio, July 27, 2021. www.michiganradio.org.

Chapter Two: Factors That Affect Mental Health

14. Quoted in Cleveland Clinic, "Does Mental Illness Run in Families?," December 2, 2019. https://health.clevelandclinic.org.
15. Quoted in Carolyn Gregoire, "Why Are Teens So Moody and Impulsive? This Neuroscientist Has the Answer," HuffPost, December 6, 2017. www.huffpost.com.
16. Caroline Fenkel, "Isolation's Silent Role in the Teen Mental Health Crisis," *Democratizing Mental Health Care* (blog), *Psychology Today*, November 3, 2022. www.psychologytoday.com.
17. Quoted in Kait Hanson, "Here's What's Really Happening on Social Media," *Today*, 2023. www.today.com.
18. Quoted in Health Matters, "Is Social Media Threatening Teens' Mental Health and Well-Being?," 2023. https://healthmatters.nyp.org.
19. Quoted in Cleveland Clinic, "Does Mental Illness Run in Families?"

Chapter Three: Recognizing Symptoms

20. Quoted in Johnson, "Defining and Understanding Mental Health."
21. Quoted in Anya Kamenetz, "A Surprising Remedy for Teens in Mental Health Crises," Hechinger Report, March 3, 2023. https://hechingerreport.org.
22. Quoted in Scripps, "Teen Depression on the Rise: What to Look For," April 25, 2022. www.scripps.org.
23. Quoted in Ginny Monk, "How Politics Derailed Mental Health Care at Killingly High School," Connecticut Mirror, August 27, 2022. https://ctmirror.org.
24. Quoted in Cleveland Clinic, "Your Child's Anxiety: When to Worry, When to Relax," July 2, 2019. https://health.clevelandclinic.org.
25. Quoted in Josie Albertson-Grove, "'Don't Stop Asking for Help': What NH Youth Are Saying About Mental Health Crisis," Seacoastonline.com, June 18, 2022. www.seacoastonline.com.
26. Quoted in Scripps, "Teen Depression on the Rise."

Chapter Four: Self-Care Strategies

27. Quoted in Maritza Moulite, "Exercise Is Good for Your Body and Your Mind, Study Says," CNN, August 8, 2018. www.cnn.com.
28. Kenneth E. Miller, "Can Taking a Break Lead to 'Aha!' Moments?," *The Refugee Experience* (blog), *Psychology Today*, March 28, 2021. www.psychologytoday.com.

29. Quoted in University of South Australia, "Exercise More Effective than Medicines to Manage Mental Health," ScienceDaily, February 23, 2023. www.sciencedaily.com.

30. Quoted in Hannah Echols, "Promote Positive Mental Health Through Back-to-School Routines," UAB News, August 8, 2022. www.uab.edu.

31. Quoted in Heather Monroe, "The Importance of Sleep for Teen Mental Health," *U.S. News & World Report*, July 2, 2018. https://health.usnews.com.

32. Quoted in Moira Lawler, "Why Friendships Are So Important for Health and Well-Being," Everyday Health, August 25, 2021. www.everydayhealth.com.

33. Quoted in USC Suzanne Dworak-Peck School of Social Work staff, "Self-Care Tips on How to Manage Stress That You Can Easily Put into Practice," USC News, April 27, 2018. https://news.usc.edu.

34. Barton Goldsmith, "The Benefits of Positive Self-Talk," *Emotional Fitness* (blog), *Psychology Today*, May 2, 2022. www.psychologytoday.com.

35. Quoted in Lynn Ma, "The Anti–Social Network: These Teens Are Ditching Instagram, Snapchat and TikTok," Chalkbeat New York, December 15, 2022. https://ny.chalkbeat.org.

Chapter Five: Reaching Out for Help

36. Quoted in Kristin Salary, "9 Reasons Why You Can Benefit from Therapy—Even If You Don't Have a Mental Illness," Insider, November 6, 2017. www.insider.com.

37. Quoted in Rob Mentzer, "Teens Talk About How They Maintain Their Mental Health," Wisconsin Public Radio, May 7, 2021. www.wpr.org.

38. Quoted in Cleveland Clinic, "Does Mental Illness Run in Families?"

39. Quoted in Kelsey Borresen, "7 Questions Your Therapist Will Probably Ask During Your First Session," HuffPost, September 9, 2019. www.huffpost.com.

40. Quoted in Jessica Truschel, "Depression Definition and DSM-5 Diagnostic Criteria," PSYCOM, August 26, 2022. www.psycom.net.

41. Quoted in Emily Torres, "How to Set (Actually Helpful) Goals for Therapy," Good Trade, September 16, 2021. www.thegoodtrade.com.

42. Quoted in Cleveland Clinic, "How To Choose the Best Child Therapy and Therapist," January 11, 2023. https://health.clevelandclinic.org.

43. Sophie Goldstone, "I Was Diagnosed with OCD at 9—by 13 I Couldn't Leave the House," Metro, March 13, 2023. https://metro.co.uk.

44. Jen Sincore Gallagher, "What Therapists Want You to Know About Mental Health," Psychology Group. https://thepsychologygroup.com.

Books

Kate Allan, *It's Your Weirdness That Makes You Wonderful: A Self-Acceptance Prompt Journal*. Coral Gables, FL: Mango, 2019.

Jennie Marie Battistin, *Mindfulness for Teens in 10 Minutes a Day: Exercises to Feel Calm, Stay Focused & Be Your Best Self*. Emeryville, CA: Rockridge, 2019.

Linette Bixby, *Mindfulness Workbook for Teens: Exercises and Tools to Handle Stress, Find Focus, and Thrive*. Emeryville, CA: Rockridge, 2020.

Barbara Diggs, *Relax: How to Manage Anxiety and Emotions in an Uncertain World*. San Diego, CA: ReferencePoint, 2023.

Janine Halloran, *Coping Skills for Teens Workbook*. Boston: Encourage Play, 2020.

Lisa M. Schab, *The Anxiety Workbook for Teens: Activities to Help You Deal with Anxiety and Worry*. Oakland, CA: Instant Help, 2021.

Internet Sources

American Psychiatric Association, "What Is Mental Illness?," 2022. www.psychiatry.org.

Elizabeth Englander and Meghan K. McCoy, "Analysis: There's a Mental Health Crisis Among Teen Girls. Here Are Some Ways to Support Them," *PBS NewsHour*, February 24, 2023. www.pbs.org.

Barton Goldsmith, "The Benefits of Positive Self-Talk," *Emotional Fitness* (blog), *Psychology Today*, May 2, 2022. www.psychologytoday.com.

D'Arcy Lyness, "I Think I Have a Mental Health Problem. Who Can I Talk To?," TeensHealth, 2022. https://kidshealth.org.

University Health Service, University of Michigan, "Ten Things You Can Do for Your Mental Health," 2023. https://uhs.umich.edu.

Go Ask Alice!

https://goaskalice.columbia.edu

The Go Ask Alice! website is a place where teens and young adults can look up information about mental, emotional, and behavioral health topics and pose questions for health professionals at Columbia University.

Mental Health Literacy

https://mentalhealthliteracy.org

This organization is a resource for teens, as well as parents, teachers, and health professionals. There is information about stress management, sleep, brain development, and many other subjects presented in accessible, easy-to-understand language.

National Alliance on Mental Illness (NAMI)

https://nami.org

NAMI is dedicated to improving the lives of people with mental illness and of their families. Its website provides information about community chapters and other resources, educational materials, personal stories of coping and thriving with mental illness, crisis intervention information, and much more.

National Institute of Mental Health (NIMH)

www.nimh.nih.gov

The NIMH sponsors mental health research and supports educational and awareness efforts across the country. Its website offers articles about dozens of mental health disorders, therapies and treatments, clinical trials, and other related news.

Substance Abuse and Mental Health Services Administration (SAMHSA)

www.samhsa.gov

SAMHSA operates the twenty-four-hour Suicide & Crisis Lifeline, and its website offers information on topics such as substance abuse, harm reduction, mental illness, mental health services in schools, and programs that intervene in cases of domestic violence, homelessness, and other issues.

Trevor Project

www.thetrevorproject.org

The Trevor Project's main goal is to end suicide among LGBTQ young people. The website offers resources on mental health, suicide prevention, and gender identity, as well as links to communicate with online counselors and connect with other young people in the LGBTQ community.

INDEX

Cover: Shutterstock.com

5: Tinseltown/Shutterstock.com
9: New Africa/Shutterstock.com
12: Image Point FR/Shutterstock.com
17: ONOKY - Photononstop/Alamy Stock Photo
21: Monkey Business Images/Shutterstock.com
24: Ground Picture/Shutterstock.com
27: Motortion Films/Shutterstock.com
31: Monkey Business Images/Shutterstock.com
34: Tero Vesalainen/Shutterstock.com
37: Neal Bryant/Shutterstock.com
40: Martin Novak/Shutterstock.com
43: Rawpixel.com/Shutterstock.com
45: Monkey Business Images/Shutterstock.com
49: VH-Studio/Shutterstock.com
53: Rawpixel.com/Shutterstock.com
55: Orion Production/Shutterstock.com